Instructor's Manual to Accompany

Introduction to Physical E
Fitness, and Sport

Third Edition

Jacalyn Lund
University of Louisville

Daryl Siedentop
The Ohio State University

Becky Berkowitz
Westerville, Ohio City Schools

Roberta Faust
The Ohio State University

Mayfield Publishing Company
Mountain View, California
London • Toronto

International Standard Book Number: 1-55934-911-5

Manufactured in the United States of America
10   9   8   7   6   5   4   3   2   1

Mayfield Publishing Company
1280 Villa Street
Mountain View, California 94041

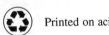 Printed on acid-free, recycled paper

Contents

True-False, Multiple-Choice, and Short-Answer Test Questions

Chapter 1

Lifespan Sport, Fitness, and Physical Education

Many students will be unaware of the degree to which sport and fitness are becoming important issues in infant education and for senior citizens. Physical education has traditionally served children and youth. Thus, a main goal for this chapter must be to provide direct or vicarious experiences for students so they can come to grips with the possibility and desirability of lifespan involvement.

True-False Questions

T 1-1 Although lifespan involvement in sport, fitness, and physical education is possible, for many people it is not yet happening.

T 1-2 People are slowly becoming exercise and diet conscious as a part of the wellness movement, which attempts to prevent illness rather than to remedy it.

F 1-3 Most school physical education programs have contributed to the fitness accomplishments of the past decade.

T 1-4 The era of muscular Christianity marked the time when many of the religious sanctions against sport and play began to diminish.

T 1-5 Organized sport did not develop to any great degree until the late nineteenth century.

T 1-6 The changes in perception and the opportunities that accompany them with regard to sport and fitness will most affect girls, women, and older people.

F 1-7 Most research indicates that enriched motor experiences for infants have no bearing on levels of adult fitness and participation in sport.

T 1-8 Early motor stimulation is a way to enrich the lives of very young children.

F 1-9 Most experts agree that sports for children are positive and beneficial.

F 1-10 Most elementary school children have physical education classes taught by a physical education specialist.

T 1-11 Most American high schools have a sports program for their students.

T 1-12 Some states have passed regulations that allow school districts to hire non-certified persons to coach sport teams.

F   1-13 Sport clubs typically cater to children's and youth sport programs.

F   1-14 Older adults tend to be the highest users of community recreation services.

T   1-15 Softball is the most popular participation sport for adults in America.

T   1-16 Young adults appear to be increasingly incorporating some aspect of sport and fitness into their lifestyle.

F   1-17 Young athletes must avoid vigorous exercise because of the damage to the heart that occurs, commonly referred to as "the athlete's heart."

F   1-18 Physical education programs now include golf and bowling so that children of today will have appropriate activities to do when they grow older.

T   1-19 Masters sport competition is for senior athletes in five-year age groups beginning at age 40.

T   1-20 Our current "senior" generation has had to learn to be active, as society did not encourage an active lifestyle when they were growing up.

T   1-21 Historically, an "athletic club" was a social club for wealthy men in a big city.

F   1-22 "Senior" women were encouraged to participate in vigorous activity during World War II, and this trend continued into the post-war years.

T   1-23 Because in the past sport, fitness, and physical education have been restricted to children, youth, and young adults, facilities have been most often associated with schools, communities, and YMCA-type organizations.

F   1-24 The private multi-purpose athletic club of today is vastly different from what has been offered by family YMCAs in the past.

T   1-25 Sports medicine centers treat and rehabilitate athletic injuries and prevent minor afflictions from becoming major problems.

F   1-26 As sport spectating increases in popularity, sport participation levels tend to decrease.

F   1-27 As sport and fitness facilities have increased in popularity, do-it-yourself exercise or exercise-at-home programs have decreased.

T   1-28 Corporation worksite fitness centers have become more common as companies have found that a healthy work force is more productive and less expensive than an unfit one.

T 1-29 Lifespan fitness should begin in early childhood so that a foundation of motor skill development can be built.

T 1-30 Physical education has traditionally reinforced the notion that there are girls' activities and boys' activities.

T 1-31 Basic skills are actually easier to develop in older children and adults because they are mentally more capable of understanding the demands of the activity.

T 1-32 Older people who see peers as activity role models will begin to see different opportunities for themselves.

F 1-33 As sport and fitness increase in popularity, the majority of jobs will be in schools where physical education programs will expand and grow.

T 1-34 The public sector has traditionally been the major source of jobs in sport, fitness, and physical education.

F 1-35 Predictions are that the public sector will expand and continue to be the primary source of jobs in the areas of sport, fitness, and physical education.

T 1-36 More and more, sport and fitness practices are attributed to scientific evidence rather than to accumulated experience.

T 1-37 As consumers of sport, fitness, and physical education become more highly educated, they will demand that the services given represent the best of what is known.

F 1-38 Physical education and fitness programs have tended to focus on the collective and structural problems of fitness in America rather than on individual fitness problems.

F 1-39 Many new professions have developed as a result of the fitness boom, all of which require preparation of the same nature as that of a physical education teacher.

F 1-40 The professions involved with sport, physical education, and fitness all require certification before an individual can obtain a job.

F 1-41 Although life expectancy hasn't increased, the quality of those years has been enhanced by physical activities.

True-False Answers

1. T	7. F	13. F	19. T	25. T	31. T	37. T
2. T	8. T	14. F	20. T	26. F	32. T	38. F
3. F	9. F	15. T	21. T	27. F	33. F	39. F
4. T	10. F	16. T	22. F	28. T	34. T	40. F
5. T	11. T	17. F	23. T	29. T	35. F	41. F
6. T	12. T	18. F	24. F	30. T	36. T	

Short Answer Questions

1-1 What is meant by lifespan involvement in activity?

ans: People become involved in purposeful activity very early in life and continue doing it throughout their lifetime.

1-2 What is the wellness movement?

ans: A movement that emphasizes prevention of sickness rather than remedy of sickness

1-3 What are the four periods which historically have seen great leaps forward in sport, fitness, and physical education? Why?

ans: a. Mid-nineteenth century: removal of many religious sanctions against sport and play
 b. Late nineteenth century: organized sport emerged in America
 c. Early twentieth century: many sport, fitness, and physical education professions developed
 d. 1960s and 1970s: the academic study of sport, fitness, and physical education emerged

1-4 What is meant by "the athlete's heart"?

ans: Vigorous exercise would cause a young person's heart to enlarge, which was thought to be detrimental.

1-5 Who is Masters sport competition for, and how is it organized?

ans: For women and men age 40 and above, organized by five-year age groups

1-6 What is school physical education like at the present time?

ans: School physical education is in a period of turmoil. It has been severely criticized by some people for its lack of accomplishment, while others recognize its importance and want to increase the time allocated for it.

1-7 What has been the traditional movement experience for a preschool child?

ans: Activities have been informally arranged and monitored, provided by parents who have had virtually no training in motor development.

1-8 What is the result of enriched motor experiences for infants and young children?

ans: They tend to be more fit and continue participation patterns into adulthood. The drive to excel may be developed and nurtured when early motor efforts are recognized and encouraged by parents.

1-9 What is a Fitnessgram?

ans: A means of communicating regular fitness test results to parents by means of a computerized printout

1-10 What are some types of activities one might see in an exemplary physical education program?

ans: a. Fitness testing and related activities
        b. Adventure skills
        c. Sports/intramurals
        d. Movement exploration

1-11 What have some school districts had to do in order to hire enough coaches for school teams?

ans: If state regulations allow, non-certified persons are hired to coach if the districts cannot find enough certified teachers to fill the vacancies.

1-12 What are some examples of how young people can compete athletically but not on a school team?

ans: a. Equestrian events
        b. Karate
        c. Ice skating

1-13 What are some ways a young adult (post high school) could be athletically involved?

ans: a. College/university intramurals
        b. City/community recreation
        c. Fitness establishments
        d. Informal (biking, jogging, walking, tennis, golf, water activities, skiing, skating, etc.)

1-14 What type of sport has traditionally been considered "appropriate" for older adults?

ans: Non-vigorous sports like golf or bowling; cycling or jogging done in a leisurely fashion

1-15 What are some "low impact" exercises in which seniors increasingly are taking part?

ans: Aerobics, walking, cycling, jogging

1-16 Contrast the historic athletic club with the one known in today's society.

ans: In the past, an athletic club was a social club for wealthy men in a big city. The modern athletic club is a place for singles, married couples, and families to participate in sport and fitness activities.

1-17 What type of organization could be considered a forerunner of a modern athletic club?

ans: YMCA

1-18 What is a sport medicine center?

ans: A place where people who participate in sport and fitness activities go for treatment, rehabilitation, remediation, and prevention of problems

1-19 What type of personnel might one find at a sport medicine center?

ans: a. Orthopedic medical specialist
        b. Family practice specialist
        c. Podiatric specialist
        d. Nutritionist
        e. Physical therapist
        f. X-ray technician
        g. Athletic trainer
        h. Sport psychologist

1-20 What has been the relationship between levels of sport participation and sport spectating?

ans: Participation and spectating tend to correlate positively; that is, as participation rates go up, so does spectating.

1-21 Why have corporations added recreation and fitness programs?

ans: Corporations have found that a healthy and physically active work force is more productive, health costs are substantially reduced, and employees tend to be more loyal to the company.

1-22 Why should the stereotype of low or no activity for senior citizens be eliminated?

ans: a. People live longer. If they are active, they will be more likely to enjoy life.
          b. Activity can decrease health care costs
          c. People with high levels of fitness will have more opportunities available to them

1-23 How will the clientele of future fitness programs be different from that of the past?

ans: a. Female as well as male
          b. Older population (more than school-age children and youth)
          c. Private facilities will service people on a larger basis than they do at present
          d. Consumers will be more knowledgeable

1-24 What issue is emerging about the type of program for the new professionals?

ans: Should the program be specialized or be of a general nature?

1-25 How will an informed private sector change the nature of physical education in the schools?

ans: a. Increased disparities between high- and low-skilled students
          b. Informed parents demanding better programs and practices

Chapter 2

The Emergence of a Profession: 1885–1930

Sport and physical education developed out of a specific historical context, which is how students should come to understand those developments. Comparing historical contextual developments with similar present developments might help to solidify and enliven their understanding. Having students provide first-person biographies of leaders and "play by play" descriptions of early events helps to heighten interest.

True-False Questions

2-1 Sport was considered to be an integral part of the physical education curriculum as it developed in the latter part of the 19th century.

2-2 The Beecher system did not win widespread acceptance because the activity was too scaled down to be of value to the women who used it.

2-3 Dioclesian Lewis published a journal in 1861, which can be considered to be the first American physical educational journal.

2-4 Hitchcock's main contribution to the growth of physical education was his emphasis on scientific measurement.

2-5 The 1889 Boston Conference could be labeled "the battle of the systems."

2-6 As late as 1850, organized intercollegiate sport did not exist.

2-7 Growth of sport interest on college campuses was largely the result of faculty and administrative effort and support.

2-8 From the earliest days of sport, college administrators were appointed to set the schedule and decide who would belong to the team.

2-9 Abuses in college athletics should be viewed as a contemporary phenomenon.

2-10 Women's intercollegiate sport has always had better controls than men's sport, and so there are fewer cases of abuse in women's sport.

2-11 Title IX has greatly increased intercollegiate sport opportunities for women.

2-12 The Chicago World's Fair Congress on Education marked the time when medicine was viewed as the parent discipline of physical education.

2-13 The conference held at the Chicago World's Fair symbolized the end of a gymnastics orientation to physical education curriculum.

2-14 The new physical education moved away from the concepts of natural play and expression in favor of a more "formalistic" approach.

2-15 Because of America's Puritan beginnings, dance was not often found in school curriculums, but gymnastics was included.

2-16 The industrial revolution of the nineteenth century created a national concern about health, especially that of children.

2-17 Fitness concerns were reflected in school curriculums along with the development of the sport culture.

2-18 The intramural programs concept began in public schools and spread slowly to colleges and universities.

2-19 If spectators attended sporting events in the early 1900s, the numbers present were typically very small.

2-20 Most early proponents of physical education had been trained as medical doctors rather than teachers.

2-21 American sports heroes and heroines emerged as Americans became more middle class and consequently had more money and time to spend on leisure.

2-22 Because there were so many draft rejections based on poor physical condition, just after World War II, most states passed laws requiring daily physical education.

2-23 According to Williams (1930), "education of the physical" is a broader view that is based on the biological unity of mind and body.

2-24 The interpretation of "education of the physical" was important because it put physical education clearly within the context of general education.

2-25 The work of Sargent and Hitchcock led to the development of a scientific emphasis in physical education.

2-26 McCloy was concerned about low fitness levels in children as the profession was forming early in the twentieth century.

2-27 The early years of growth and development of physical education were clearly dominated by the thoughts and work of white males.

2-28 The American Civil War temporarily halted the development and standardization of many sport forms.

2-29 Muscular Christianity made exercise and fitness compatible with Christian life and thus helped set the stage for the development of physical education.

2-30 New England Puritanism helped to expand the philosophies of sport and play, which explains why so many important developments occurred in this section of the country.

2-31 Physical education, as we know it, was largely European in its development.

2-32 The early YMCA movement used sport and exercise to reach and serve youth, thus helping to reduce religious opposition to these concepts.

2-33 Sport was actually a mechanism by which early immigrants could be Americanized.

2-34 The industrial revolution led to long working hours and little free time, thus slowing the growth of sport and fitness.

2-35 The intellectual climate present during the nineteenth century contributed to the growth of sport and fitness, as change was the theme of the century and maintaining status quo was not.

2-36 Title IX has retarded the growth and expansion of sport as more monies had to be channeled to female athletics.

2-37 Today's track and field activities would typically be associated with a Swedish exercise system.

2-38 The Swedish exercise system was associated with a developmental and therapeutic emphasis, using both active and passive exercise patterns.

2-39 Sargent's system consisted of exercise machines, Swedish and German type exercises, and calisthenics.

2-40 Basketball and volleyball are both American sports that evolved from European forerunners.

True-False Answers

1. F	7. F	13. T	19. F	25. T	31. F	37. F
2. F	8. F	14. F	20. T	26. T	32. T	38. T
3. T	9. F	15. F	21. T	27. T	33. T	39. T
4. T	10. T	16. T	22. F	28. F	34. F	40. F
5. T	11. T	17. T	23. F	29. T	35. T	
6. T	12. F	18. F	24. F	30. F	36. F	

Short Answer Questions

2-1 What is "muscular Christianity"?

ans: A philosophy that made exercise and fitness compatible with Christian life

2-2 What were the virtues attributed to women during the nineteenth century?

ans: Piety, purity, submissiveness, and domesticity

2-3 What happens when a sport becomes standardized or institutionalized?

ans: a. Rules become standard
     b. Bodies are formed to enforce those rules
     c. Standards of competition are set
     d. The sport is promoted for both participants and spectators
     e. Championships are formed
     f. Records are kept
     g. Traditions and rituals are developed

2-4 What controls did early athletic conferences invoke on participants?

ans: a. Eligibility requirements for new students
     b. Eligibility requirements for students while participants
     c. Limitations on athletic aid
     d. Limitations on how coaches were hired and retained

2-5 What meeting symbolized the fact that physical education was a legitimate subject?

ans: The International Congress on Education held at the Chicago World's Fair in 1893

2-6 What were the four phases of the educational process Hetherington felt should be considered in physical education?

ans: a. Organic education
          b. Psychomotor education
          c. Character education
          d. Intellectual education

2-7 What system was associated with a *turnplatz*? What does *turnplatz* mean?

ans: The German System. A *turnplatz* was an outdoor gymnasium or exercising ground.

2-8 What sport transition do historians say occurred during the thirty years following the American Civil War?

ans: Sports were transformed from local games to institutionalized sport.

2-9 As religious prohibitions against exercise and fitness began to relax, what other concept, important to our profession, started to be accepted?

ans: The idea that exercise and fitness were educationally important

2-10 What impact did immigrants have on sport and physical education?

ans: They brought with them new games and attitudes. Sport became a mechanism through which they became Americanized.

2-11 How did the urbanization movement in America lead to the development of sport?

ans: Americans could not conveniently hunt, fish, and pursue other outdoor activities as in the past, and sport grew to fill that void.

2-12 Briefly describe the intellectual climate of the mid-nineteenth century and its subsequent influence on sport and physical education.

ans: It was a time for new ideas, and the status quo was in flux. Because of all this change, new concepts were more readily accepted than in the past, and the ideas of sport and physical education—although quite different from the rather conservative past—were really not that dramatically unique.

2-13 In the early gymnastics systems, what is meant by the "formal approaches to exercise"?

ans: Formal meant that the movements were prescribed and done in unison by a group of students.

2-14 What two important elements contributed to the popularity of the various exercise systems?

ans: a. Loyalty to the gymnastics system was in many ways tied to loyalty to a given country
       b. The dominant psychology of that time sought to train the mind by doing precise, repetitive, and orderly activities

2-15 How were the German and Swedish systems the same and how did they differ?

ans: Both used an apparatus system on which to do exercises and were implemented to build stronger individuals and to instill a sense of national pride. The Swedish System tended to have more of a developmental-therapeutic emphasis, whereas the German System was of a more running and track and field nature. The Swedish System also included passive exercises wherein a therapist manipulated the patient.

2-16 What was the motivation behind the Beecher system of gymnastics?

ans: That the typical gymnastics system for men was too vigorous and required too much strength for women

2-17 Describe the Dio Lewis gymnastics system.

ans: It was less vigorous than the German System yet vigorous enough to increase the heart rate. Music accompanied the exercises, which were graceful and flowing.

2-18 How did German politics contribute to the growth of the "German" gymnastics system?

ans: A failed revolution in Germany led to a flood of German immigrants to America. The system was popular because it signaled a pride in the country.

2-19 Which system had a scientific basis because of its emphasis on measurement?

ans: The Hitchcock System

2-20 What was the relationship of sport and games to the various "systems"?

ans: Sport and games were not fundamental to any of these systems and at that time had no place in physical education.

2-21 What sport is considered our first national sport, and when did it become a national sport?

ans: Baseball, which spread rapidly during and after the Civil War

2-22 How did education in America differ from the classical European models?

ans: The classical European models of education were designed for the upper class, whereas Americans were pursuing the concept of a universal public education.

2-23 In the nineteenth century, what was the educational background of most physical education leaders, and what did this mean for the physical education curriculum?

ans: Most were prepared as medical doctors, and the curriculum emphasized formal gymnastics in which hygiene and fitness were important outcomes.

2-24 What educational theories replaced those of formalism?

ans: Natural play and expression

2-25 Who developed the Universal Test for Strength, Speed, and Endurance?

ans: Dudley Sargent

2-26 In 1918, a commission sponsored by the National Education Association (NEA) identified seven principles as national goals for education. What are two that had a direct bearing on the field of physical education?

ans: a. Health
        b. The worthy use of leisure time

2-27 What effect did the contributions of Edward Hitchcock and Dudley Sargent have on the American gymnastic systems as compared to their European counterparts?

ans: American programs had a much more scientific basis than the European ones.

2-28 Compare how golf, football, and basketball differ with their introduction into American sports history.

ans: Golf was introduced into America in essentially the same form as that played in Europe. Football is a variation from a sport that has European roots, but now football is a unique American product. Basketball was created by an American and had no previous European counterpart.

2-29 The Puritan work ethic and absence of a substantial "gentleman" class have been cited as reasons for abuse in early collegiate sport. How did these two quite different concepts contribute to this abuse?

ans: The Puritan work ethic was that there was a job to do and one did everything possible to achieve that end (win). The lack of a gentleman class put few restraints on how that goal was accomplished. Winning within the rules became lost to the philosophy of winning at any cost.

Chapter 3

Consolidation and Specialization: 1930–Present

The contextual nature of developments should be emphasized, perhaps by attempting to forecast future developments based on the trends developed in this historical period. "Game show" formats are good ways to identify leaders, important personalities, and events of this period. How the events of this period have affected the sport and fitness experiences of your students—forms of activity, opportunities, etc.—is a good entry to making the history more personally relevant.

True-False Questions

3-1 The 1929 Carnegie Report was generally favorable toward the advances and growth of collegiate sport.

3-2 The budget cuts mandated by the Depression led to the first-ever elimination of physical education from the curriculum because of its "frill" nature.

3-3 Recreation programs increased in popularity during the Depression.

3-4 During Depression years, the wealthy were the only people able to participate in sports/recreation programs.

3-5 Many national and state parks were built during the Depression by the Civilian Conservation Corps.

3-6 During the Depression, the Works Progress Administration was responsible for the construction of gymnasia, swimming pools, ski facilities, and stadiums.

3-7 The professional organization for physical educators merged with the NEA, changing its name to the American Association for Health and Physical Education.

3-8 The curricular model advocated by the LaPorte monograph (1938) was used only briefly by physical educators.

3-9 World War II moved the goal of fitness back into the physical education curriculum, as soldiers were found to be basically unfit for the rigors of war.

3-10 Recreational sports such as badminton, archery, and table tennis were not often played by soldiers during World War II because more vigorous, fitness-promoting activities were encouraged.

3-11 Physical education was not considered a "frill" subject during World War II but rather a vital part of a school curriculum.

3-12 Physical education motor learning research had its early beginnings in World War II, when airplane gunners needed to be trained.

3-13 Rehabilitation of soldiers injured in World War II led to the field of adaptive physical education.

3-14 The Kraus-Weber tests brought the fitness status of American children to the attention of political leaders.

3-15 The Kraus-Weber tests were measures of cardiovascular and muscular endurance.

3-16 Because he was a sports fan and enjoyed playing touch football, John F. Kennedy began the President's Council on Youth Fitness.

3-17 Physical educators responded to the call for improved youth fitness by making fitness the dominant theme of their program.

3-18 In 1954, *Brown v. the Topeka Board of Education* eliminated the separate but equal concept that allowed schools to be segregated on the basis of race.

3-19 Wilderness sport and adventure education has direct ties to American consciousness of pollution and environmental concerns.

3-20 Title IX was aimed primarily at better opportunity in sport and physical education for minority racial groups.

3-21 Public Law 94-142 was the legislation designed to ensure the rights of handicapped Americans.

3-22 Although two generations ago athletes typically specialized in one sport, now they often receive the benefits of cross training by participating in two or three sports.

3-23 The Olympics have increasingly differentiated between amateur and professional athletes.

3-24 In general, Americans have had no underlying concern about the lack of fitness until recent times, when fitness has become fashionable.

3-25 Fitness promotion in the private sector has led to greatly improved physical education programs.

3-26 Since the recent emphasis on fitness in the general culture, experts no longer are strongly concerned about the fitness levels of children.

3-27 The academic reform movement that followed Sputnik resulted in an increased emphasis on competition in physical education.

3-28 The growth of scientific activity in the discipline of physical education led to an emphasis on knowing what was happening as opposed to merely doing an activity.

3-29 Adventure physical education allows students the opportunity to participate in activities in the natural environment.

3-30 Although movement education is highly popular in England, its goals and values have never been widely accepted in the United States.

3-31 Title IX has accounted for few curricular changes in physical education, but sports teams have been greatly affected by it.

3-32 As the number of doctoral degrees granted in physical education increased, the research base expanded as well, creating a context favoring the discipline approach to physical education.

3-33 Legislation in California contributed to the expansion of the physical education discipline movement.

3-34 The most well-developed research area early in the discipline movement was motor development.

3-35 The subdisciplines in physical education have tended not to associate closely with the parent discipline, preferring to work exclusively within the field of sport.

3-36 The American Association of Health, Physical Education, and Recreation changed its structure to conform with the discipline movement by becoming an Alliance so as to encompass all related areas.

3-37 The discipline of sport pedagogy was begun as a means of accommodating the subdiscipline of teacher education.

3-38 As sport pedagogy research developed, most teacher education programs quickly incorporated that knowledge base into their programs.

3-39 States have preferred to control education of physical education teachers, so attempts to standardize education at a national level have not been considered important issues.

3-40 Fitness was not a major issue in society during the Depression but did become so when World War II began.

3-41 As a result of the War Fitness Conference in 1943, school physical education was encouraged to teach sport activities to provide recreation for soldiers home on leave.

3-42 The availability of monies for research projects contributed greatly to the physical education discipline movement.

True-False Answers

1. F	7. T	13. T	19. T	25. F	31. F	37. T
2. T	8. F	14. T	20. F	26. F	32. T	38. F
3. T	9. T	15. F	21. T	27. F	33. T	39. F
4. F	10. F	16. F	22. F	28. T	34. F	40. T
5. T	11. T	17. F	23. F	29. T	35. F	41. F
6. T	12. T	18. T	24. T	30. F	36. T	42. F

Short Answer Questions

3-1 List three programs from the Depression era that had a direct impact on sport fitness and physical education.

ans: a. Civilian Conservation Corps
   b. Works Progress Administration
   c. National Youth Administration

3-2 What two things stymied the growth of collegiate and professional sport during the late 1920s and early 1930s?

ans: a. The Great Depression
   b. The 1929 Carnegie Report about abuses in collegiate athletics

3-3 What was the major influencing factor on the growth of sport in the 1950s and 1960s?

ans: Television

3-4 Why was the attention given to physical fitness in the 1950s and early 1960s so important?

ans: It showed the relationship of physical fitness to health and cardiovascular disease.

3-5 What has helped to partially reconceptualize the role of women in society?

ans: The growth of women's sports

3-6 What has been estimated to be the largest youth program for boys and girls?

ans: Soccer

3-7 What is a type of exercise popular in today's fitness landscape?

ans: Aerobic fitness

3-8 Who was responsible for the beginning of the discipline movement in physical education?

ans: Franklin Henry

3-9 What was the status of physical education during the Depression?

ans: It was considered a frill subject and was cut from school budgets.

3-10 During the Depression, interest shifted from spectator to participatory programs. What related field increased substantially?

ans: Recreation

3-11 What is considered America's most popular recreational sport?

ans: Softball

3-12 What curriculum model was advocated in the LaPorte Monograph (1938)? Briefly describe the model.

ans: A "block" or "unit" approach was advocated wherein activities were offered for periods of time lasting three to six weeks. The basic plan gave time for initial instruction and some skill development and culminated in game play.

3-13 Why wasn't fitness the focus of society during the Depression?

ans: Basic needs for food, shelter, and employment overshadowed fitness in importance.

3-14 What event brought the issue of fitness back to prominence?

ans: With the beginning of World War II, many inductees failed physical tests and had trouble with the physical aspects of basic training.

3-15 What happened to the status of physical education during the early 1940s?

ans: It was once again considered an important part of the school curriculum and outlived the frill status it experienced during the budget cuts of the Depression.

3-16 Why are the beginnings of motor learning traceable to the war effort?

ans: Many war skills were really motor skills and visual discrimination skills. For example, training for airplane gunners and aircraft lookouts involved motor skills.

3-17 Why did adapted physical education begin in World War II?

ans: Thousands of wounded soldiers needed both rehabilitation and activities in which they could experience satisfaction from leisure participation.

3-18 What impact did the Kraus-Weber tests have on physical education?

ans: Sports and leisure sports had been the primary topics of physical education. The Kraus-Weber tests made fitness a national priority for the next decade and beyond.

3-19 What did the Kraus-Weber tests measure?

ans: Flexibility and strength of the lower back

3-20 How did Rachel Carson's book affect physical education?

ans: The growth of wilderness sport and adventure education has direct ties to environmentalist themes of this era.

3-21 What was Title IX of the Education Amendments?

ans: A congressional action through which girls and women might finally have equal access to sport and fitness

3-22 What was the main focus of Public Law 94-142?

ans: It was designed to ensure the rights of persons with disabilities, especially in education.

3-23 How have ideas about "working out" changed over the past twenty years?

ans: Going to a gym to work out would have meant a smelly place with poor facilities. Today going to a fitness center is almost a social event. Being fit is fashionable and very socially acceptable.

3-24 What are triathlons?

ans: Competitions in which participants run, swim, and bike

3-25 Following the Sputnik reforms in education, what was the counter movement found in physical education?

ans: Competition was downplayed in favor of cooperative activities. New games, martial arts activities, and adventure sports were added to curriculums.

3-26 What type of adventure skills can be taught on the school site with a slight modification of school facilities?

ans: Climbing and rappeling

3-27 What was the Fisher Act, and why was it significant for physical education?

ans: A bill passed in California that required all departments to have an academic base. It caused physical educators to redefine the field as an academic discipline rather than as an applied program.

3-28 What were the early subdiscipline areas that developed as a result of the discipline movement?

ans: a. Biomechanics
      b. Motor learning
      c. Sport psychology
      d. Sport history
      e. Sport philosophy

3-29 What positive characteristic has been a result of the discipline movement and its parent disciplines?

ans: Bridges have been built linking the subdiscipline of those trained in physical education with those trained in the parent discipline.

3-30 What reorganizing move did AAHPER make in 1973 so as to continue being an umbrella over the various disciplines?

ans: AAHPER changed its name from "association" to "alliance" in an effort to minimize the splintering that inevitably occurred as the subdisciplines formed their own groups.

3-31 How did teacher education programs react to the discipline movement?

ans: They felt that, although the disciplines were important, they did not replace the learning of sport skills and the acquisition of teaching skills. A new subdiscipline representing teacher education called sport pedagogy was formed.

3-32 Give several examples of how sport grew and expanded during the years following World War II.

ans: a. NFL, Major League baseball, and NBA expansion
          b. Golf
          c. Olympics
          d. Collegiate sport
          e. Youth sport

3-33 What is the current label used to describe programs that are disciplinary based, and what organization has decided to use that label?

ans: Kinesiology; the American Academy of Kinesiology and Physical Education

Chapter 4

Changing Philosophies for Sport, Fitness, and Physical Education

Philosophies are highly contextual; i.e., they need to be understood in terms of the historical period in which they were prominent. Thus, this chapter should be related to Chapters 2 and 3. All students will have personal philosophies; the material in this chapter should serve to help them further articulate and evaluate their own points of view. Relating historically important philosophies to current movements can be helpful, such as the relationship of the current fitness movement to our medical beginnings, the current feminist movement to the masculine/feminine expectations of the nineteenth century.

True-False Questions

4-1 Nationalism was the common idea that gave rise to both the German and Swedish gymnastics systems.

4-2 Because of the group dynamics of the Swedish and German gymnastics systems, which fit well with military training concepts, both of the systems were limited to the health and well-being of the state.

4-3 The early Puritans used play as a means for getting the body fit to better serve God.

4-4 Ralph Waldo Emerson played a significant role in the development of the muscular Christian philosophy.

4-5 The idea that participation in sport had moral benefits was in nearly complete concurrence with Puritan beliefs.

4-6 Muscular Christianity espoused the virtues of fitness for males but not necessarily for females.

4-7 In muscular Christianity, women were encouraged to participate in and watch sports, rather than pursue fitness goals.

4-8 In the late nineteenth century, being an amateur in sport typically meant that one was from a wealthy family and was highly coached by those most knowledgeable about the sport.

4-9 As Pierre de Coubertin revived the Olympics, the emphasis placed on winning led to their rapid growth and intense levels of competition.

4-10 Because of the need for child labor, John Dewey's educational agendas included attempts at making children more mature at an earlier age.

4-11 Dewey believed that education should be an active experience and that doing was equally important as knowing.

4-12 Dewey advocated physical education, especially when applied to achievement of social goals.

4-13 Jean-Jacques Rousseau supported physical education because he believed cooperation and competition could be fostered through that medium.

4-14 Early educators such as Pestalozzi and Froebel emphasized the cognitive aspects of education with little concern for the physical.

4-15 Wood and Hetherington's goals for "education through the physical" stood in stark contrast to the ideas professed by Pestalozzi and Froebel.

4-16 As progressive education gained support, play became a legitimate and important focus for education.

4-17 With the rise of Christianity, play was viewed negatively, as work was the desired form of activity for virtuous people.

4-18 Philosophies accepting the concept of play were crucial before programs advocating play could be implemented.

4-19 The growth of the physical education movement was retarded somewhat because those prominent in physical education were not influential in other fitness, playground, and YMCA movements.

4-20 The predominant philosophy of the first half of the twentieth century professed that children learn most naturally by playing.

4-21 The philosophy of "education through the physical" has remained unchallenged and firmly in place through the present time.

4-22 Rudolph Laban is associated with the development of the human movement philosophy.

4-23 Because the human movement philosophy exists harmoniously with that of "education through the physical," human movement has been widely accepted by most physical educators.

4-24 Physical education teacher education departments had difficulty justifying the academic nature of their programs when relying solely on the "education through the physical" philosophy.

4-25 The human movement philosophy, which advocates an exploratory approach to teaching physical education, has been most popular at the secondary level.

4-26 Human movement philosophy emphasizes the development of sport skills along with the movement related to these skills.

4-27 Body awareness, space, and qualities of movement are concepts utilized in movement education as a basis for understanding all movement.

4-28 Academic specializations in physical education recently have begun to rely on the human movement philosophy to tie them together.

4-29 The two major educational movements of the post-Sputnik era were the renewed emphasis on science and mathematics and the human movement philosophy.

4-30 In humanistic education, personal and social development of the child is at least as important as academic development.

4-31 Humanistic education has remained a popular movement in educational circles, especially in conjunction with the conservative 1980s.

4-32 The goal of play education was to help students acquire skills as well as an affection for the activities themselves.

4-33 Proponents of play education consider physical education equal to the other institutionalized forms of play: drama, art, and music.

4-34 Play education promotes physical education for its social, emotional, and moral benefits.

4-35 Advocates of sport education feel that the development of good sport persons and a better sport culture should be central to the goal of physical education.

4-36 In sport education the students participate in a sport for an extended time (season) and go through a competitive schedule that has a championship at its conclusion.

4-37 The growth of the wellness concept has closely paralleled the fitness boom.

4-38 Freedom from disease would be an adequate definition of the wellness concept.

4-39 Wellness is an individual responsibility and, therefore, should be approached primarily through an individual's education.

4-40 The wellness/fitness movement was first found in public schools and later spread to the private sector, as business people realized the huge profits available.

True-False Answers

1. T		7. F		13. T		19. F		25. F		31. F		37. T
2. T		8. F		14. F		20. T		26. F		32. T		38. F
3. F		9. F		15. F		21. F		27. T		33. T		39. F
4. T		10. F		16. T		22. T		28. F		34. F		40. F
5. F		11. T		17. T		23. F		29. F		35. T		
6. T		12. T		18. T		24. T		30. T		36. T		

Short Answer Questions

4-1 How did the Victorian Age's stereotype of women prevent them from participating in vigorous sports activities?

ans: Vigorous exercise and competitive sports were generally thought to be inappropriate for women.

4-2 How did masculine stereotypes contribute to the difficulty in changing the feminine stereotype?

ans: Men had to be tough, virile, and aggressive. American men were accused of becoming too feminine. To keep males masculine, girls had to remain feminine.

4-3 Trace the chain of influence, explaining the links, from Rousseau to Dewey.

ans: *Rousseau* wanted an education to be natural, with the individual growing up in perfect freedom. He believed humans were created good and were ruined by contact with society. Rousseau believed the mind and the body were interrelated.

Basedow put Rousseau's natural educational philosophy into practice. In his school, sensory learning was dominant. Children used natural objects in their learning. Children were treated as children rather than as miniature adults.

Pestalozzi felt sensory learning was the keystone of educational methodology, so great importance was placed on physical training of all kinds, physical labor as well as gymnastics, sports, and games. Pestalozzi wanted unity in the child, harmony in the intellect and heart.

Froebel believed in the unity of life and the unity of action that was expressed in observing, creating, discovering, and exercising. He was a strong advocate of physical play and felt that sports and games developed students' physical talents, strengthened their intelligence, and developed their character.

Dewey was influenced by the ideas of Froebel.

4-4 What was the accepted mode of behavior through which children learned most naturally during the first half of the twentieth century?

ans: Play

4-5 Describe the human movement philosophy.

ans: It advocates a more open, exploratory approach to teaching physical education. In movement education, all activities are selected on the basis of how well they can foster and develop the concepts and movement principles described under body awareness, space, and qualities of movement. These concepts or elements of movement became the framework of a movement education curriculum.

4-6 List the four areas of development considered important for youth in the first half of the twentieth century that could be achieved through physical education.

ans: a. Intellectual
        b. Moral
        c. Physical
        d. Social

4-7 What fundamental concept provided the linkage from Rousseau to Dewey?

ans: Play

4-8 What are the institutionalized forms of play?

ans: a. Art
        b. Music
        c. Drama
        d. Physical education

4-9 What two branches form the speculative branch of philosophy?

ans: a. Metaphysics
        b. Axiology

4-10 The critical branch of philosophy comprises:

ans: a. Epistemology
        b. Logic

4-11 What was the common idea that gave rise to the European exercise systems?

ans: Nationalism, a pride in one's country

4-12 What philosophy was known for its stern view of human life, which left little room for physical activity not related to work and took a harsh view of anything that was playful?

ans: Puritanism

4-13 Which American philosopher provided great impetus for moving toward a muscular Christian philosophy?

ans: Ralph Waldo Emerson

4-14 Describe the philosophy of muscular Christianity.

ans: Physical fitness and sporting prowess were important avenues through which mental, moral, and religious purposes were developed and sustained.

4-15 During the Victorian Age, what was the status of exercise for girls and women?

ans: While mild forms of "proper" exercise were thought to be useful, vigorous exercise and competitive sports were generally thought to be inappropriate, because it might be harmful and it promoted behavior that was unladylike.

4-16 Who were the amateur sport participants? Describe their typical training regimen.

ans: Being an amateur in sport typically meant you were male and rich. They did not train full time, nor did they receive any real coaching.

4-17 Why would the motto of the Olympics have seemed out of place in ancient Greece?

ans: In ancient Greece, only the winner of Olympic contests won prizes. The motto downplays the importance of winning, recognizing instead the importance of participation.

4-18 What was the progressive education theory?

ans: In progressive education, doing was as important as knowing. Students were actively involved in learning instead of being passive recipients of knowledge. The unity of man was important, so the physical as well as the cognitive aspects were taught.

4-19 Why did Rousseau advocate physical education in the schools?

ans: He felt games and sports were important in developing cooperation and competition.

4-20 Who was responsible for the creation of the human movement philosophy?

ans: Rudolf Laban

4-21 When university physical education departments were forced to justify the academic nature of their programs, the "education through the physical" philosophy gave way to what movement?

ans: The discipline movement

4-22 What ideas are professed by the humanistic or third force psychology?

ans: The personal, social development of children was thought to be more important than, or at least as important as, academic development. Open education, affective education, values clarification, and less emphasis on competition for grades and academic outcomes are all part of this philosophy.

4-23 What happened in the world of sport around the same time that humanistic philosophy gained popularity?

ans: Several books were written that condemned the abuses in sport, criticized how athletes were treated, and advocated reforms.

4-24 What is the current status of the humanistic movement in physical education?

ans: It did not survive the 1970s, as the nation turned more conservative in the 1980s.

4-25 What was the goal of play education?

ans: To acquire skills and an affection for the activities themselves

4-26 What do the number of community theaters, the weekend golfer, and a member of a music group all have in common?

ans: Each is at play, only the form differs.

4-27 What is the current status of the play education movement?

ans: Play education never became a reality because it was more a philosophy than a prescription for a program.

4-28 How did the philosophy of play education influence the curriculum?

ans: Physical educators began to be more aggressive in arguing that their subject matter was valuable in and of itself. It did not need to be justified by reference to objectives or outcomes outside the subject matter.

4-29 What was the purpose of sport education?

ans: To educate students in the skills, values, and attitudes of good sport so that they might enjoy and participate themselves and also want to be active contributors to a healthier sport culture

4-30 On what rationales is sport education based?

ans: a. Sport derives from play
         b. Sport is important in our culture
         c. If sport is a higher form of play, and if good sport is important to the health and vitality of the culture, then sport should be the subject matter of physical education

4-31 How would a sport education unit (season) be designed?

ans: a. Students are on a team for an entire season
         b. A schedule of competition is established
         c. A culminating event or season finale is arranged
         d. Records are kept
         e. Traditions are developed

4-32 What economic classes are involved in the fitness movement?

ans: Middle and upper classes

4-33 What does the wellness movement profess?

ans: Being free from disease and pain as well as being active and in good spirits

4-34 How does a nation achieve wellness for more of its citizens?

ans: By educating about wellness and providing opportunities to practice wellness so that race, socioeconomic condition, or gender are not barriers.

Chapter 5

Basic Concepts of Sport

The concept of play is typically difficult for students. Try having them observe different play groups: children at recess, high school students on a basketball court, a junior high sport team. The different meanings of competition are nearly always a good entry to exploring students' points of view. A nationally televised contest is always a good way to "catalog" the rituals associated with sport as a natural religion.

True-False Questions

5-1 Most scholars agree that sports are institutionalized forms of play.

5-2 According to anthropologists, all people, everywhere, play in one form or another.

5-3 Using Caillois's characteristics of play, when sport is "free," there are no costs for participating or watching.

5-4 Sport is most playful when it is uncertain, meaning that the participants had no idea that the game was to begin prior to its actual start.

5-5 To the extent that new wealth is produced, the playfulness of the activity decreases.

5-6 In keeping with the playful nature that underlies all sport, sport, by definition, has to be playful.

5-7 Play can be viewed as a necessary aspect of behavior that requires no justification or further explanation.

5-8 Developmental psychologists believe that children acquire much of their early knowledge about the physical and social world through play.

5-9 All play should have the characteristics of turbulence, gaiety, spontaneity, and diversion.

5-10 Adult play tends to put emphasis on practice, skill, and strategy.

5-11 Adult play devises obstacles that make it more difficult and increase the challenges.

5-12 As sport loses the characteristics of playfulness, the meaning increases for the participants.

5-13 Using Loy's definition, all games are sport.

5-14 Although some scholars differentiate games from contests (e.g., swimming or marathon running), the activities are so similar that each can be referred to as a game, as defined by Loy (1969).

5-15 By definition, a non-competitive game cannot exist.

5-16 Chess, bridge, and board games are considered sports even though they involve no physical skill.

5-17 Any game can be made more developmentally appropriate by altering its primary rules.

5-18 A 30-second shot clock in basketball or a 45-second time between plays in football are examples of secondary rules.

5-19 Territory games are those in which each team has a territory defined and the other team cannot cross that line (example: volleyball, badminton).

5-20 Basketball and ice hockey are target games.

5-21 Frisbee is not considered a game, as it has not been institutionalized.

5-22 Competition is almost always defined as a rivalry in which opponents strive to gain something at the expense of others.

5-23 Zero-sum competition is a unique form of rivalry where opponents must tie the score before the game is completed.

5-24 Pursuit of competence seems to be a more consistent motivator for young athletes than rivalry, the most frequently associated meaning for the word *competition*.

5-25 The rivalry aspect of competition does not always include another individual or team; it also can mean the competition against an ideal standard or record.

5-26 When much importance is attached to winning and losing in sport, the play element in competition is greatly enhanced.

5-27 When a game has a common form that can be recognized anywhere, the game is said to have become institutionalized.

5-28 Many professions develop as a role becomes institutionalized, to the point that their number is greater than those actually playing.

5-29 Since sport is meaningful only when it is a fair contest, the referee's main role is to ensure that neither opponent gains unfair advantage by violating the rules.

5-30 The most competent officials are needed at the least institutionalized games/sports so that the growth and development of the activity can be consistent and fair.

5-31 The institutionalization of sports has led to the development of specialized jobs and professions such as sport management and sport promotion.

5-32 Records in sport are one way that excellence is defined and preserved.

5-33 Research shows that the primary motivation for continued participation by young people is to strive for increased competence.

5-34 Although young athletes may know what some of the records are in their sports, successful coaches will not emphasize these to avoid discouraging young athletes.

5-35 Sport emerged as an important part of our culture concurrently with the development of communication technologies.

5-36 Most sport spectators enjoy the entertainment aspects of the game but are not actually very knowledgeable or sophisticated as viewers.

5-37 Because the factors that influence the development and popularity of sport in a culture affect both participation and spectating, as more people participate in a sport, more tend to watch it as well.

5-38 Although all sport can be said to contain some aesthetic components, the competition, rather than beauty or grace, remains the most important factor.

5-39 As sport in America developed, so did the philosophy of fair play, which puts Americans at a disadvantage when competing at the international level.

5-40 The beauty of a gymnastic routine has higher aesthetic value than does a well-executed fast break in basketball.

5-41 Rules that can be violated to gain a competitive advantage are bad rules because they eliminate the evenness of the game.

True-False Answers

1. T	7. T	13. F	19. F	25. T	31. T	37. T
2. T	8. T	14. T	20. F	26. F	32. T	38. T
3. F	9. F	15. T	21. T	27. T	33. T	39. F
4. F	10. T	16. F	22. T	28. T	34. F	40. F
5. T	11. T	17. F	23. F	29. T	35. T	41. T
6. F	12. F	18. T	24. T	30. F	36. F	

Short Answer Questions

5-1 What is thought to be the motivating impulse underlying the development of drama, art, and music?

ans: Play

5-2 What are the six characteristics of play according to Caillois?

ans: a. Free
      b. Separate
      c. Uncertain
      d. Economically unproductive
      e. Governed by rules (regulated)
      f. Make believe (fictive)

5-3 What are the six characteristics of adult play?

ans: a. Practice
      b. Training
      c. Rituals
      d. Costumes
      e. Skill
      f. Strategy

5-4 What is Loy's definition of a game?

ans: Any form of playful competition whose outcome is determined by physical skill, strategy, or chance, employed singly or in competition

5-5 Why is the term "non-competitive game" a contradiction?

ans: Without some element of competition, the activity would cease to be a game.

5-6 What are the four classifications of sport, based on similarities among the primary rules?

ans: a. Territory or invasion games
         b. Target games
         c. Court games
         d. Field games

5-7 List the five types of rivalry.

ans: a. Team vs. team
         b. Individual vs. individual
         c. Individual vs. a previous best performance
         d. Individual vs. a physical barrier
         e. Individual vs. a record

5-8 In what ways could sport be considered to be like a religion?

ans: There are rituals, vestments, a sense of powers that are outside one's control, those that can enforce the rules and mete out punishments, and role models. Sport also teaches such admirable qualities as perseverance, courage, and sacrifice.

5-9 What are the characteristics of children's play?

ans: a. Turbulence
         b. Gaiety
         c. Spontaneity
         d. Diversion

5-10 What are the characteristics of adult play?

ans: a. Calculation
         b. Subordination to rules
         c. Contrivance
         d. Ritual

5-11 Give examples of obstacles that adults could add to play to make a game more challenging. The following are examples of possible answers:

         a. Shooting archery from a greater distance
         b. A more challenging golf course with sand traps, water holes, narrow
             fairways, etc.
         c. Playing basketball with better opponents
         d. Singles tennis instead of doubles

5-12 Explain the difference between primary rules and secondary rules.

ans: Primary rules of a game identify how the game is to be played and how winning can be achieved. Primary rules are what make basketball basketball and not volleyball.
        Secondary rules can be altered or modified to make the game developmentally appropriate or different in some way without changing the essential characteristics of the game.

5-13 Identify and explain the four categories of sports as determined by their similarities among primary rules.

ans: a. Territory or invasion games are defined by the problem of needing to invade the space of the opponent in order to score.
        b. Target games are defined by the primary rules of propelling objects with great accuracy toward targets.
        c. Court games are defined as strategically propelling an object in ways that cannot be returned by an opponent.
        d. Field games are defined by primary rules that require one opponent to strike an object in such a way as to elude defenders on the field.

5-14 What must happen to an activity before it is considered to be a sport?

ans: It must become institutionalized, which means that there are standardized rules to which all players adhere, a governing body for the sport, and a growing sense of traditions associated with the sport. A common form of the game is needed with primary rules.

5-15 What is zero-sum competition?

ans: What is gained by one competitor must be lost by the other competitor.

5-16 What are the three meanings that competition can have?

ans: a. Coming together: the festival aspects of competition
        b. Competence: striving to achieve an objective or to become competent
        c. Rivalry: striving to gain something at the expense of others

5-17 What two things determine how people play the game and what is expected of them?

ans: a. Rules
        b. Traditions

5-18 Why are intentional rule violations looked upon with disfavor by those concerned with ethics and the true nature of the game?

ans: Intentional fouls are violations of the spirit of a contest. When one player or team purposely tries to use the rules to gain an advantage, they are changing the nature of the test, without the consent of their opponent.

5-19 Why does the play of a child typically change to the adult end of the continuum?

ans: That way of playing appeals more to a mature person and has better sustaining power.

5-20 What is sport?

ans: Sports are games that involve combinations of physical skill and strategy.

5-21 Why aren't games of chess and dice considered sport?

ans: Games of dice involve chance as a primary determinant of the outcomes. Chess involves strategy but no physical skill. Since sports are games that involve combinations of physical skill and strategy, neither would be considered sport.

5-22 What two aspects of competition do researchers say are most motivating for young athletes?

ans: a. Getting better in their sport (competence motivation)
b. Festival characteristic (affiliation with the sport)

5-23 What factors will seriously diminish the play element in sport?

ans: a. Uneven opponents
b. Required participation
c. Economic consequences
d. Pressures for winning that carry over to "real" life

5-24 What is the relationship of the number of sport professionals to the level of institutionalization of a sport?

ans: The lower the level of organization, the fewer the professionals. A sandlot game only needs participants but as the game becomes more organized, a coach is added. This increasing complexity continues until at professional levels of sport, related professionals outnumber the participants.

5-25 What is the main role of the referee?

ans: To ensure fairness by seeing that all contestants honor the rules and that no contestants get an advantage that is disallowed by the rules

5-26 What must be ensured before a record can be part of a sport?

ans: The competition must be fair, using standard rules and good officiating.

5-27 What become standards through which young athletes define their improvement?

ans: Records by which their progress and potential can be defined and charted. These records will be for the individual and compared with those of others in their own competitive bracket as well as those of elite athletes.
        In sports where records are not kept, the athlete tests himself or herself directly against the competition.

5-28 What is one of the clearest indications of the new level of seriousness with which sport is examined?

ans: The growing number of sports literature books

5-29 What is the relationship between sport participation and sport spectating?

ans: The more people participate in sport, the more watch it

5-30 According to Novak, in what way are sports spectators participants?

ans: The mode of observation proper to a sports event is to participate or extend one's own identification to one of the sides and "join the team," in a sense.

5-31 What are form sports?

ans: When the physical form of the performance is the determining factor in the competition

5-32 According to Carlisle, what are the four types of aesthetic quality which can be present in sport?

ans: a. The beauty of a well-developed body in motion
        b. The beauty of a brilliant play or a perfectly executed maneuver (more intellectual than physical)
        c. The beauty of the dramatic nature of sport competition
        d. The beauty of the unity achieved by an athlete or a team throughout a competition

5-33 What is the philosophic study of values called?

ans: Axiology

5-34 How does the tradition of fair play differ from the "win at all costs" approach to sport competition?

ans: Within the tradition of fair play, the primary goal of sport is victory within the letter and spirit of the rules. To win at all costs violates this philosophy. It is not possible to win if the rules are broken, because that changes the game.

5-35 What is the purpose of a penalty?

ans: To restore evenness to the contest, to provide for the offended player or team some measure that makes up for what they lost because of the offending action

Chapter 6

Sport Programs and Professions

It's always interesting to "localize" the major concepts in this chapter. What kinds of sport are done for different age groups? Who organizes it? Who pays for it? What full- or part-time jobs are locally available? How much do people earn in those jobs? How are local school coaches paid? What are participation rates? How do the opportunities divide between public and private? Visits (or reports from visits) to local clubs and facilities can be useful.

True-False Questions

6-1 Americans have less leisure time than the ancient Greeks and Romans.

6-2 The work week of today is longer than those in most other historical periods.

6-3 Career people (e.g., doctors, lawyers, business executives) tend to have more free time than blue-collar workers.

6-4 Sport is a leisure activity pursued mainly by those seeking to fill free time.

6-5 A player who participates on a softball team in a league would be classified as a recreational participant.

6-6 A non-professional may make money from his or her participation but may draw on that money only to cover living expenses.

6-7 Youth sport throughout the world tends to be funded by private agencies rather than by the government.

6-8 Little League baseball as well as YMCA and YWCA programs are supported in part by funding from the federal government.

6-9 Children and youth of all ages and skill levels have open access to sport leagues and programs in the United States.

6-10 Youth coaches in the United States usually have had training in sport but little formal preparation in pedagogy.

6-11 Countries with governmental involvement in youth sport programs require different levels of training for various levels of competition.

6-12 Because education in the United States is provided for in the Constitution, organization of school sport is, in essence, controlled by the federal government.

6-13 The total numbers of interscholastic sport participants have dropped in recent years, indicating the negative influence of television and video games.

6-14 The growth of women's volleyball in interscholastic competition is largely the result of Title IX legislation.

6-15 Interscholastic sport is typically governed by a state agency that is usually a part of the state department of education.

6-16 Schools are required by law to pay for all extra-curricular activities, including costs for interscholastic competition.

6-17 Although there is variation for coaching requirements from state to state, all states do require a teaching certificate or coaching certification.

6-18 Coaching certification usually requires coursework in the science area classes, certification in first aid, and study in coaching theory.

6-19 The United States is still the only country in the world where sport and college/university education are so intricately linked.

6-20 The National College Athletic Association (NCAA) and the National Association of Intercollegiate Athletics (NAIA) are both organizations affiliated with the federal government.

6-21 Larger schools tend to affiliate with the NCAA.

6-22 Junior colleges (two-year schools) are not affiliated with NCAA or NAIA.

6-23 The main purpose of professional sport is to provide an outlet for outstanding talent while at the same time providing enjoyment for millions of fans.

6-24 Once an athlete achieves professional status, a lucrative income will accompany the position.

6-25 The average length of a professional career is usually 4 to 6-1/2 years.

6-26 A professional sports team usually will have as many non-participant professionals as professional athletes.

6-27 Professional sports are governed mainly by the owners as opposed to any type of federal affiliation.

6-28 Low levels of recreational league participation accentuate the point that we are a nation of spectators rather than doers.

6-29 Most people cite social and competitive experience as their reason for league participation.

6-30 Public Law 94-142 required a free and appropriate public education for people with disabilities, including the area of physical education.

6-31 Disabled persons have more than thirty national sport organizations from which to select an area of interest or an area that best fits their needs.

6-32 Special Olympics are restricted to disabled children of school age.

6-33 Masters sports competition is for those age thirty and above who still desire to compete in athletics.

6-34 Sport management/administration programs require many internship hours and business courses but few courses in the physical education field.

6-35 A good athletic trainer is certified and deals exclusively with injuries and rehabilitation.

6-36 Athletic trainers need certification, which can require from 400 to 1800 hours of clinical experience.

6-37 Minority persons are frequently found in non-participant sport professions as well as in participant-performer roles.

6-38 With the advent of Title IX, the number of women in coaching and administrative roles has substantially increased over the past decade.

6-39 Sport managers feel that the competencies most important to their profession are human relations, personnel management, time management, and writing.

6-40 Many professional leagues are instituting recruitment and development programs to increase the number of minority persons in coaching and administrative positions.

6-41 The three main foci for sport management careers are intercollegiate/professional sport, sport/recreation industries, and health/fitness industries.

True-False Answers

1. T	7. F	13. F	19. T	25. T	31. T	37. F
2. T	8. F	14. T	20. F	26. T	32. F	38. F
3. F	9. F	15. F	21. T	27. T	33. F	39. F
4. F	10. T	16. F	22. T	28. F	34. T	40. T
5. F	11. T	17. F	23. F	29. T	35. F	41. T
6. T	12. F	18. T	24. F	30. T	36. T	

Short Answer Questions

6-1 Which peoples historically worked as many days as they played or had festivals?

ans: Greeks and Romans

6-2 List four characteristics of youth sport programs that nurture healthy physical, psychological, and emotional growth and development.

ans: a. Fun and enjoyable for the participant
        b. Foster moral sensitivity and caring
        c. Exercise a spirit of discovery, adventure, and creativity
        d. Inspire a sense of community

6-3 What are the four participation categories for sport?

ans: a. Recreational participant
        b. Amateur athlete
        c. Non-professional athlete
        d. Professional athlete

6-4 What are two organizational features of sport for children and youth in the United States?

ans: a. Not funded by the government
        b. Tends to be exclusionary for older youth

6-5 What are the four ways recreational sport in America is sponsored?

ans: a. Community recreation departments
        b. Business or industry
        c. Service clubs
        d. Private community organizations typically started and maintained by parents

6-6 What are the two reasons most people compete in recreational leagues?

ans: a. Social experience
        b. Competitive experience

6-7 What does NATA stand for?

ans: National Athletic Trainer Association

6-8 How does the work week of today compare with that from other historical periods?

ans: It is probably longer.

6-9 What is happening to the length of the average work week for factory and service industry workers?

ans: It is getting longer.

6-10 What is a non-professional athlete?

ans: An athlete who may make money from his/her participation but may draw on that money only to cover living expenses and keep the remainder in escrow until retirement

6-11 What is the average beginning age for competitive sport?

ans: 11

6-12 What is the purpose of the "Parent's Checklist for Quality Youth Programs" (NASPE, 1995)?

ans: Provides a series of statements to help parents evaluate the developmental and educational benefits likely to accrue from children's and youths' participation in any sport program.

6-13 In the United States, for youths age 13–18, where is the primary place for sport participation?

ans: The schools

6-14 Why is interscholastic sport organized and regulated at the state level with little or no federal input?

ans: In the United States Constitution, education is specifically designated as a state function.

6-15 Why has the number of interscholastic sport participants in the United States declined?

ans: There are fewer students, as the baby boom generation is no longer in school.

6-16 What are some of the ways interscholastic sport is funded?

ans: a. Tax revenues through regular school budgets
        b. Gate receipts, fund raisers, booster club
        c. Students pay directly to play

6-17 What piece of legislation has created a substantially greater need for coaches? Why?

ans: Title IX. More girls are participating in sport.

6-18 Why do qualifications for coaching vary among the states?

ans: The governance of education is left to the states by the United States Constitution.

6-19 Which is the only country in the world where sport and college/university education have become so completely linked?

ans: The United States

6-20 What determines the NCAA division to which schools belong?

ans: a. Level of competition
        b. Rules for financial aid to athletes

6-21 What types of sports exist for disabled athletes?

ans: Disabled persons can do virtually every sport that fully able persons do.

6-22 List five nonparticipant sport professions.

ans: Sport management, athletic training, sport broadcasting, sport publicity, officiating, sport psychology, sport journalism, etc.

6-23 What are the main components of the undergraduate sport management program?

ans: General education, courses in sport management, and work experiences

6-24 What are the two main paths to certification in athletic training?

ans: Completion of a formal program or an internship program

Chapter 7

Problems and Issues in Sport

It is easier to get students to discuss some problems (appropriate/inappropriate competition for children) than others (sex equity). Formal debates or panels responding to specific issues can help to initiate further discussion and comment. It is interesting to compare participant views on problems to those of coaches/administrators. Developing an ideal community youth program or an ideal school program is often an entry to get students thinking about improvements.

True-False Questions

7-1 Good competition should manifest the characteristics of play—e.g., be even, voluntary, and strictly governed by rules.

7-2 Good competition should be arranged so that fans and spectators can be entertained and enjoy what they are watching.

7-3 For competition to be appropriate, the rules and equipment should reflect the developmental characteristics of the competitors.

7-4 Pressures or support from coaches and parents make up the largest part of what is called the psychological climate of children's sport.

7-5 Cooperation, while necessary in team sports, is not a major issue in individual sports.

7-6 Research on young athletes has shown that competence, affiliation, and fun are more important enduring motivations for participation than winning.

7-7 Most scientific experts suggest that children should not begin organized sport before the age of fourteen.

7-8 The social and psychological abilities necessary to cooperate with teammates and compete against others in a game is typically underdeveloped prior to age eight.

7-9 Because young children cannot understand the concepts of competing, young children should not participate in skill development programs or programs that have any elements of loosely organized competition.

7-10 The epiphysis is vulnerable to injury because of a limited blood supply and limited healing potential.

7-11 Play can be more likely to cause epiphyseal injuries than youth sport because without adult supervision, children tend to continue to play even when they feel pain.

7-12 Children who are put on weight training programs as the result of youth sports are less susceptible to injury.

7-13 To be most fun and useful for children and youth, sports need to be modified to be developmentally important.

7-14 When games are modified for children and youth, they are safer and therefore more desirable, but they are not as exciting for the participants.

7-15 Youth of today tend to concentrate and train for a single sport, whereas athletes of the past tended to participate in several sports.

7-16 Overuse injuries have tended to decrease with sport specialization.

7-17 Students who specialize in sports are more likely to experience burnout than a three-sport athlete.

7-18 Youth coaches are typically viewed in a favorable manner because of their knowledge of the game and because they provide much corrective feedback and evaluation of players' performance.

7-19 In the Coach Effectiveness Program, winning is important, but it is not the only goal of a program.

7-20 Research has shown that negative interaction patterns are typically associated with lessened achievement and lowered self-concepts.

7-21 The three major amateur sports organizations in America, the NCAA, the U.S. Olympic Committee, and the Amateur Athletic Union, are involved in coaching education and have helped to enhance both children's and youth sport.

7-22 Children typically would rather sit on the bench with a winning team than play actively on a losing team.

7-23 Pressures applied to youth that make winning a game or contest important outside that context, greatly diminish the playful nature of competition.

7-24 The Aussie Sport Program is an example of how the government can work with the corporate sector for the improvement of sport experience for children.

7-25 The varsity model of competition makes sport increasingly available to youth as they get older.

7-26 The European club system tends to be exclusionary as youth get older, only making provisions for elite athletes.

7-27 Although the total number of injuries in football is decreasing, the number of serious injuries has continued to rise.

7-28 Most school sports are relatively free from injury, largely due to the rules associated with training and competition.

7-29 Injuries associated with sports other than football tend to be from inadequate weight training and are most frequently found in athletes who participate in several sports and who thus fail to strengthen those specific areas most needed for the sport in which they are currently involved.

7-30 In Division III schools in the NCAA, no scholarships are given for athletic prowess.

7-31 Drug testing for college athletes may be unconstitutional under the Fourth Amendment, which prohibits unreasonable search and seizure.

7-32 The vast majority of NCAA Division I athletic programs are supported by gate receipts from their football and basketball programs.

7-33 Pay to play plans will negatively impact large suburban schools more than inner-city schools' interschool sports programs.

7-34 When considering the hours an athlete spends "working" for his or her athletic scholarship, the pay per hour is lower than minimum wage.

7-35 In many respects, the Olympic Games held in ancient Greece were ahead of their time because they allowed for the participation of females in events such as archery and running.

7-36 In spite of Title IX, in many places girls' teams do not have equality in the use of facilities, travel to games, uniforms, or equipment.

7-37 Research indicates that signs of assertiveness in young girls are now accepted and encouraged.

7-38 After Jackie Robinson broke the "color barrier" in major professional sport, top level intercollegiate sport quickly followed suit and integrated its ranks as well.

7-39 Problems of race in sport tend to interact with economic issues, as the more affluent have better access to instruction.

7-40 Nowhere in the world is school or university sport as important to a sport culture as in the United States.

7-41 The United States has increased its governmental support for athletics to a level equal to that (per capita) of the support given in other countries.

7-42 Schools that have not complied with the provisions of Title IX have been vigorously prosecuted.

True-False Answers

1. T	7. F	13. T	19. T	25. F	31. T	37. F
2. F	8. T	14. F	20. T	26. F	32. F	38. F
3. T	9. F	15. T	21. F	27. T	33. F	39. T
4. T	10. T	16. F	22. F	28. T	34. T	40. T
5. F	11. F	17. T	23. T	29. F	35. F	41. F
6. T	12. F	18. F	24. T	30. T	36. T	42. F

Short Answer Questions

7-1 What is the four-part philosophy of the Coaching Effectiveness Training?

ans: a. Winning isn't everything, nor is it the only thing; that is, winning is an important goal but not the only goal.
b. Failure is not the same as losing; therefore, losing need not imply personal failure in any way.
c. Success is not synonymous with winning; therefore, winning doesn't relate directly to sense of personal triumph any more than losing does to personal failure.
d. Success is found in striving for victory and is related to effort as much as or more than to outcome.

7-2 List the three things that research indicates children would choose about their sport experience.

ans: a. Want to play rather than watch
b. Sports should be modified so they can play better
c. Less emphasis from the outside to win

7-3 What has been the recent focus of *Sport for All* programs?

ans: Physical fitness, especially that of worksite programs for employees

7-4 The state where the athlete is simply tired of doing the same thing over and over for years in a row is called

ans: Burnout

7-5 What name is given to the school sport model used in the United States where sport is decreasingly available to youth as they get older?

ans: Varsity

7-6 What two developments in sport have led to the tendency of sport specialization?

ans: a. Value and importance of weight and endurance training have been recognized
      b. More athletic scholarships

7-7 What are the major problems associated with school sport?

ans: a. The exclusionary or "varsity" model of interscholastic sport
      b. Injuries
      c. Eligibility and pass to play rules
      d. Specialization in sport
      e. The teacher/coach role conflict
      f. Parental pressures

7-8 List the major issues and problems found in intercollegiate sport.

ans: a. Recruiting violations and pressures
      b. Drugs to enhance performance
      c. Economic disparities among top powers
      d. Economic pressures for winning
      e. Treatment of athletes while at the university

7-9 What are the major problems and issues associated with child and youth sport?

ans: a. Premature entry into organized sport (when children are too young)
      b. Overuse injuries
      c. Sports that are developmentally inappropriate
      d. Specialization
      e. Lack of training of coaches
      f. Outside pressure for winning from coaches and parents
      g. Children and youths dropping out of sport programs
      h. Unequal access based on socioeconomic status

7-10 What two things were indicated by the scrutiny and criticism of sport?

ans: a. Sport had become vitally important in the culture.
        b. There was an "underside" to sport that needed to be attended to, or the sport culture might weaken.

7-11 What injury occurs in children that has serious developmental consequences?

ans: The epiphyseal injury

7-12 What makes any competition good and appropriate?

ans: a. The rules must respect the developmental characteristics of the participants.
        b. The psychological climate of the competition must be developmentally appropriate.
        c. It should manifest the characteristics of play.
        d. The participants are bound up in a cooperative effort learning lessons in cooperation as well as competition.

7-13 According to the experts, why shouldn't children begin organized sport before the age of eight?

ans: The social-psychological abilities necessary to cooperate with teammates and compete with them in games is typically undeveloped prior to age eight.

7-14 In what type of sport programs should children younger than age eight participate?

ans: Skill-oriented programs that have elements of loosely organized competition

7-15 According to teaching research, what effect does negative interaction have on achievement and self-concept?

ans: Negative interaction patterns are *always* associated with lessened achievement and lowered self-concepts.

7-16 How does the European system differ from the United States interscholastic model?

ans: The European Club System gives youths the opportunity to learn and compete based on interest. The United States varsity model provides opportunity only for those skilled enough to make the team.

7-17 According to a NATA survey, briefly discuss the incidence of injury in football.

ans: The total number of injuries is decreasing. The number of serious injuries is increasing.

7-18 What body part is the most vulnerable in football?

ans: The knee

7-19 What types of injuries are most common in sports other than football?

ans: Moderate injuries—mainly overuse injuries

7-20 What appears to be the greatest hope for future control of injuries?

ans: More knowledgeable coaches and athletic trainers

7-21 What is the Aussie Sports adjunct program SPORTFUN?

ans: It is an after-school program targeting unsupervised elementary-school children. Instruction is provided by trained high-school students who work under the supervision of teachers.

7-22 What problem arises when too much pressure is put on the student athlete?

ans: The sport experience can rapidly become less than it should be.

7-23 Why do Division III schools have fewer problems with athletics?

ans: No scholarships are given for athletic prowess. Nobody expects the sports to pay for themselves.

7-24 What pressures usually lie behind recruiting violations?

ans: Economic factors as well as the status that is awarded to those associated with winning programs at universities

7-25 What are anabolic steroids?

ans: Male hormones that help to increase strength and allow athletes to perform more work in training

7-26 What legal controversy exists over drug testing?

ans: Drug testing is done to ensure that athletes have not gained an unfair advantage by using illegal drugs. There is a question as to whether testing is legal or if it violates the Fourth Amendment, which prohibits unreasonable search and seizure.

7-27 In terms of competitors, how were the ancient Olympic Games like those of 1896?

ans: The competitors were males and tended to be of a privileged/wealthy class.

7-28 Give some examples of how athletic prowess in women is still not widely accepted.

ans: a. Unequal use of facilities and budgets
        b. Sports announcers referring to a female athlete as pretty when this has nothing to do with the competition
        c. Assertiveness not being reinforced or accepted for girls

7-29 How does the funding of sport in most of the rest of the world differ from that in the United States?

ans: The overall system elsewhere is funded by the government. In the United States, funding comes mostly from the private sector.

7-30 What is the main general goal of the *Sport for All* program?

ans: Participation

7-31 What are the names and countries of some of the national *Sport for All* programs?

ans: a. Trim; Norway
        b. Life Be In It; Australia
        c. Deportito; Mexico

7-32 What is the most recent focus of *Sport for All* type programs?

ans: Physical fitness, working especially toward the development of worksite fitness programs

7-33 Describe the importance of the epiphysis in development. Why are epiphyseal injuries so serious in young children?

ans: The epiphysis is a secondary growth center. Injury to this area risks permanent injury or disability. There is a limited blood supply to this area, thus limited healing.

7-34 Identify and explain the three reasons given for epiphyseal injuries in children's and youth sport.

ans: a. When left alone, children typically quit when they feel pain; adults sometimes will encourage participation despite the pain.
    b. Children specialize in a sport today on almost a year-round basis, stressing bones in the same way and leading to overuse injuries
    c. Children are put in weight training programs in which physical stresses. produce epiphyseal injuries.

7-35 In what ways can sports be modified so that they are more developmentally appropriate for youth? Give examples.

ans: a. Equipment can be modified.
    b. The size of the field can be changed.
    c. The length of the game or contest can be modified.
    d. The rules are changed so that they respect the developmental characteristics of the participants.

7-36 Explain the three purposes modifications to games serve.

ans: a. They allow younger participants to develop skills more quickly and efficiently.
    b. The changed game is more exciting, fun, and rewarding to the participants.
    c. Rules can be developed to ensure that all participants have equal opportunities to learn and play the sport.

7-37 Discuss the problems (bad news) of youth coaches as well as the good news. What can contribute to the negative behavior seen from youth coaches?

ans: Bad news: They typically behave in ways that are not productive for young athletes; too much evaluation, too many corrective feedback statements, too many negative interactions, too few supportive interactions
    Good news: They can change!

7-38 What are the positive and negative issues associated with eligibility rules in high school sport?

ans: If school sport is "extracurricular," then it is a privilege to be earned. If school sport has basic educational value, then the opportunity for development should be available to all students. Athletes typically have to meet eligibility requirements more stringent than those necessary for a student to remain in school.

7-39 What is the teacher/coach role conflict?

ans: A person has a given amount of energy and time. Teaching is often not given as much of these as coaching is. Conflict arises when one of these roles suffers at the expense of the other.

7-40 What are some factors that contribute to pressure on a school sport participant?

ans: a. Playing in front of a crowd
        b. Write-ups in newspapers
        c. Parental and/or coach pressure
        d. The school wants a winner

Chapter 8

Basic Concepts of Fitness

A typical group of students will have *done* most of what is covered in this chapter, although some of the technical concepts may be new. Having students report on specific strength or endurance motor performance training systems will help. More difficult will be the examination of myriad health fitness approaches. A good assignment is for students to bring in evidence (magazines, newspapers, etc.) of health fitness myths, such as "miracle" programs.

True-False Questions

8-1 Our understanding of what it means to be fit has improved over the past four decades, and measurement of this fitness has become much more specific.

8-2 Evidence from exercise epidemiology suggests that high levels of regular physical activity are related to lowered death rates.

8-3 The components of health fitness are general in that everyone should achieve and maintain them.

8-4 Motor performance fitness for a golfer would be defined differently than that for a basketball player.

8-5 Health fitness is related more to reducing the risk of degenerative diseases than to better sport performance.

8-6 Without question, the most serious of the infectious diseases are associated with the heart and cardiovascular system.

8-7 When body fuels are metabolized through exercise in the presence of oxygen, this is an aerobic activity.

8-8 For national health goals, motor performance fitness is as important as cardiovascular fitness.

8-9 The relative percentage of fat, muscle, and bone that makes up body weight is called body composition.

8-10 Power is the ability to perform movements repeatedly and quickly.

8-11 Threshold of training is the intensity, frequency, and duration of exercise necessary to cause improvement in a specific component of fitness.

8-12 Aerobic exercise can help reduce percentage of body fat, reduce blood pressure, and increase insulin sensitivity.

8-13 Lower back problems are considered degenerative diseases and can be remediated with appropriate strength exercises.

8-14 The socioecological view of fitness focuses on the structures in society that promote or prevent various groups from participating in healthy lifestyles.

8-15 Motor performance fitness is related to prevention and remediation of degenerative diseases.

8-16 People's concerns with how they look, their cosmetic fitness, is not a positive part of the overall fitness movement.

8-17 The major significant difference between athletes today and their counterparts a generation ago is in amount of strength.

8-18 In sport, strength needs to be developed for a specific purpose rather than as a general phenomenon.

8-19 The "dose-response debate" refers to the level of performance-enhancing aids one can take to improve sport performance.

8-20 Increasing the energy potential of the muscle cell is the primary goal emphasized in training for fitness.

8-21 ATP must be generated from either the aerobic or anaerobic breakdown of energy, as none is stored in the cell.

8-22 ATP can be produced aerobically from the breakdown of muscle glycogen.

8-23 The lactic acid system activates with exercise periods lasting between ten seconds and three minutes.

8-24 Lactic acid is the by-product of fat and carbohydrate breakdown.

8-25 Persons whose activity patterns classify them as "least fit" are 3–4 times more likely to die earlier than people who are classified as "most fit."

8-26 Training will actually increase the number of capillaries per muscle fiber.

8-27 An unfit person uses less oxygen during maximum exertion than an elite athlete.

8-28 The principle of progression means that a sufficiently high stress must be placed on a muscle for it to require adaptation.

8-29 Muscles will atrophy and decrease in size if stresses are applied to them below what they can handle.

8-30 Large increments in stress or resistance will allow the muscles to be overloaded and show training effects faster than if small increases in load are used.

8-31 In a trained athlete, the higher the intensity of exercise, the less time is needed for rebuilding and recovery.

8-32 If exercise is of long duration, more time is needed for rest and recovery.

8-33 Distance runners should allow at least a day of recovery time whereas weight lifters could lift every day.

8-34 The target heart rate of a thirty-year-old individual working at a typical training threshold is 133 beats per minute.

8-35 To achieve maximum aerobic benefit as training progresses, the intensity or speed of running should be constant as the duration or distance is increased.

8-36 Daily workouts are necessary for health fitness purposes.

8-37 The "no pain, no gain" view of health fitness is inappropriate.

8-38 Anaerobic and aerobic training have equal value for health fitness.

8-39 Anaerobic training is used by athletes who want to perform at maximal intensities for short periods of time, as in sprinting, wrestling, and football.

8-40 To build muscle endurance, one would do few repetitions with high resistance.

8-41 A 5RM weightload is generally thought to be about 75% of maximum for most individuals.

8-42 A weightload at or exceeding 75% of one's maximum lifting capacity is most beneficial for developing and maintaining strength.

8-43 Joint flexibility can be decreased if a weight lifter fails to exercise the muscle or muscle group through the full range of motion.

8-44 A weight machine is designed so that the raising phase provides all of the desired benefits.

8-45 A weight lifter can create strength imbalances if both agonist and antagonist muscles are not utilized equally.

8-46 Accumulating 30 minutes per day of moderate to vigorous physical activity is sufficient to produce important health benefits.

8-47 Body composition is a better indicator of health fitness than weight.

8-48 MVPA takes into account a more narrow range of physical activities than did health-related aerobic fitness.

8-49 An "interpretation zone" approach to the assessment of fitness provides a means to interpret norm-referenced scores.

8-50 In the socioecological view of fitness, a person's physical activity patterns are viewed as their individual responsibility.

True-False Answers

1. T	9. T	17. T	25. T	33. F	41. F	49. F
2. F	10. F	18. T	26. T	34. T	42. T	50. F
3. T	11. T	19. F	27. T	35. T	43. T	
4. T	12. T	20. T	28. F	36. F	44. F	
5. T	13. T	21. F	29. T	37. T	45. T	
6. F	14. T	22. F	30. F	38. F	46. T	
7. T	15. F	23. T	31. F	39. T	47. T	
8. F	16. F	24. F	32. T	40. F	48. F	

Short Answer Questions

8-1 Historically, what classification of disease has been the primary source of health problems for humans?

ans: Infectious disease

8-2 Why are heart and vascular system diseases called "the cardiovascular plague"?

ans: During the last fifty years, they have become the leading cause of death in the United States.

8-3 Define muscular strength and endurance.

ans: The ability to continue successive exertions under conditions where a load is placed on the muscle groups being used

8-4 Define cardiovascular endurance.

ans: The ability to maintain effort when demands are placed on the functions of circulation and respiration

8-5 Define muscular power.

ans: The ability to release maximum force in the shortest period of time

8-6 Define flexibility.

ans: The degree of range of movement at specific joints and in total body movement

8-7 Define speed.

ans: The ability to make successive movements of the same kind in the shortest period of time

8-8 Define agility.

ans: The ability to change positions in space

8-9 Define balance.

ans: The maintenance of equilibrium while stationary or moving

8-10 Define accuracy.

ans: The ability to control voluntary movements toward an object

8-11 What are the health fitness components?

ans: a. Cardiovascular endurance/capacity
         b. Flexibility
         c. Body composition
         d. Muscular endurance
         e. Strength

8-12 What are the components of motor performance fitness?

ans: a. Coordination
        b. Agility
        c. Power
        d. Strength
        e. Balance
        f. Reaction time
        g. Speed

8-13 What are diseases that are caused by or related to a lack of appropriate physical activity called?

ans: Degenerative or hypokinetic disease

8-14 What are the diseases associated with hypokinetic disease?

ans: a. Coronary heart disease
        b. High blood pressure
        c. Low back pain
        d. Obesity
        e. Diabetes
        f. Osteoporosis

8-15 What are the three sources of ATP?

ans: a. A small amount is stored in the muscle
        b. It can be produced anaerobically from muscle glycogen
        c. It can be produced aerobically from the breakdown of carbohydrates and fats

8-16 What are the two ways body fat can be measured?

ans: a. Skinfold calipers
        b. Hydrostatic weighing

8-17 What three factors represent the threshold of training or the training effect?

ans: a. Intensity
        b. Frequency
        c. Duration

8-18 What factors are debated when experts argue the dose of activity necessary to produce health benefits?

ans: a. What activity
         b. For how long at a time
         c. At what intensity
         d. How frequently

8-19 In reference to aerobic fitness, identify the components that must become fit and what they mean for enhanced performance.

ans: The heart muscle must be fit to pump large amounts of blood. Blood must be capable of carrying large amounts of oxygen. Arteries must be free and not restrict the flow of blood. Muscles must be capable of using the oxygen to make ATP. The more fit the components, the better able the athlete will be to enhance the performance.

8-20 Explain the principles of overload, progression, and recovery time.

ans: *Overload* When one puts enough stress on a muscle for it to require adaptation. The muscle must get stronger.
    Progression Where large increments in stress or resistance are avoided because they will result in injury or chronic fatigue.
    Recovery time The time the body needs for rebuilding and recovery, without which it will break down.

8-21 How does a weight lifter's training differ for building muscle endurance and muscle strength?

ans: To build muscle endurance, one would perform numerous repetitions against a fairly low resistance. To build muscular strength, one would perform few repetitions against a much higher weight.

8-22 What is the socioecological view of health fitness?

ans: The view that structures in society promote or prevent access to healthy lifestyles based on gender, race, and socioeconomic status

8-23 What is the difference between norm-referenced fitness standards and criterion-referenced health standards?

ans: Norm-referenced standards are based on the performance of a population, while criterion-referenced health standards are based on the level of functioning necessary to maintain health.

8-24 Define power.

ans: The ability to generate force at a fast rate of speed, typically over a short distance (Force × Distance × Speed)

8-25 What is the importance of health fitness?

ans: It can help to prevent and in some cases remediate degenerative disease.

8-26 What does the "social gradient" in health and longevity refer to?

ans: Social class influences behaviors in important risk factors which lead to increasing health problems and shorter lives.

8-27 Of what benefit is motor performance fitness?

ans: It will enable a person to perform motor tasks better and more efficiently.

8-28 What component of motor performance has made a significant difference between athletes of today and their counterparts a generation ago?

ans: Strength

8-29 Why is the training program for a wrestler different from a basketball player's?

ans: Different muscles are utilized with different requirements placed on them; training for a sport needs to be specific to that sport.

8-30 How is cosmetic fitness related to health fitness?

ans: Cosmetic fitness involves looking fit and looking strong but should not be confused with health-related fitness.

8-31 How does one feel when lactic acid starts to build up after exercise? What type of exercise causes this to happen?

ans: One feels out of breath; the muscles tighten up and burn. High-intensity activities usually from one to three minutes in length are the type of exercise associated with this.

8-32 What three methods have been used to interpret the results of fitness assessments?

ans: a. Norm-referenced standards
        b. Criterion-referenced standards
        c. Interpretation zones

8-33 How does recovery time differ for weight lifters and distance runners?

ans: High-intensity exercise requires more rebuilding and recovery time. Weight lifters should put a day of rest between exercise sessions, whereas distance runners could exercise daily.

8-34 What type of training is necessary for those interested in health fitness?

ans: Aerobic exercise

8-35 Calculate the target heart rate for a thirty-year-old person exercising at a typical intensity.

ans:
$$\begin{array}{r} 220 \\ \underline{-30} \\ 190 \\ \underline{\times.7} \\ 133 \end{array}$$

8-36 What frequency is sufficient to develop and maintain high levels of health fitness?

ans: Three to five times per week

8-37 What is interval training?

ans: A means of training for an endurance event where exercise bouts are interspersed with rest periods

8-38 Which type of fitness benefits from anaerobic training?

ans: Motor performance fitness

8-39 What four primary variables must be considered in strength training?

ans:
    a. The amount of resistance (weight)
    b. The number of repetitions each time lifted (a set)
    c. The number of sets per workout
    d. The number of workouts per week

8-40 What is a 10RM load and what does it represent?

ans: This is the most weight one could lift ten times in succession and is generally thought to be about 75% of one's maximum lifting capacity for most individuals.

8-41 What is the most common form of cardiovascular function testing?

ans: Max VO$_2$ test on a motor driven treadmill

Chapter 9

Fitness Programs and Professions

Localizing (see Chapter 6) can again be helpful. Most fitness programs will have publicity brochures, and a collection of those can help. Reports of visitations can provide vicarious experiences. Serious attention should be given to local wage rates in these programs. The availability of ACSM or YMCA certification should be explored. If many students are headed for teacher certification, an interesting question to explore is "Why can't school fitness programs be more like clubs?"

True-False Questions

9-1 The death rate from degenerative disease among persons who have an inactive lifestyle is twice that of those who exercise regularly.

9-2 Estimates are that approximately 80 percent of adults in America do not get enough exercise to develop and maintain adequate health fitness.

9-3 The fitness boom is most prominent in lower socioeconomic families.

9-4 Increased family incomes as well as the women's movement have contributed to the growth of fitness participation.

9-5 Throughout history, fitness tests have evaluated the health fitness components of youth.

9-6 The 1985 National Youth Fitness Survey assessed elementary age children in grades K–4.

9-7 The primary measure of cardiovascular fitness in the National Youth Fitness Survey was an 800 meter run.

9-8 The NCYFS II showed that children carry more body fat than is healthy and do poorly on tests of upper body strength.

9-9 Inactivity is as great a risk factor for hypokinetic disease as smoking is.

9-10 Most children get sufficient physical activity daily to meet ACSM guidelines.

9-11 About 50–60% of boys participate on interscholastic sport teams.

9-12 As adults get older and have fewer demands on their time, participation in regular exercise seems to increase.

9-13 Nearly 25% of all American children can be classified as obese.

9-14 Lack of time was one of the most frequently noted reasons for non-participation.

9-15 Blue-collar workers and professional persons tend to participate in sports activities more frequently than do white-collar workers.

9-16 The NCYFS II survey showed that children in the mid-1980s carried less body fat than did their predecessors 20 years earlier.

9-17 Participation rates for girls are less than those for boys in most fitness studies.

9-18 The 1987 resolution, introduced in the United States Senate, promoting daily physical education has been instrumental in leading to increased time requirements for physical education in the schools.

9-19 School programs that focus on physical fitness occur, for the most part, outside physical education class time.

9-20 The main reason that employee fitness has become popular in the corporate sector is for the tax incentives offered by the government.

9-21 Success of employee fitness programs usually depends on the allocation of company time for fitness and facilities being available.

9-22 Employee fitness programs tend to be more available for management and administrative personnel than for other workers.

9-23 Norm-referenced fitness standards allow you to compare yourself to a population that is unfit.

9-24 The President's Council on Youth Fitness was established in 1956 when American children showed inferior fitness levels to European children through a battery of tests.

9-25 The majority of children receive physical education in elementary school from a specialist teacher.

9-26 The Fitnessgram is a joint venture of the American Heart Association and AAHPERD that promotes cardiovascular fitness via rope jumping activities.

9-27 In older age groups, frequent fitness participation has declined in the past few years.

9-28 The AAHPERD has provided leadership by offering a national certification for fitness instructors.

9-29 The CDCP Guidelines rely heavily on involving children and youth in community physical activity programs.

9-30 The ACSM has created six levels of certification that require written exams, practical experience, and in most cases CPR training.

9-31 The YMCA has an intensive certification program that, when completed, represents the level of preparation an undergraduate physical education major would have.

9-32 An undergraduate degree in exercise science is typically designed to prepare the young professional for a role in the realm of adult or corporate fitness or fitness programming.

9-33 A person obtaining a degree as a fitness major would take many of the same courses as a physical education teacher but would focus on the business aspects of fitness rather than acquiring teaching skills.

9-34 Most graduate degrees in fitness require a good background in science coursework and usually require 12–24 months to complete.

9-35 The most difficult problem associated with fitness is getting people to change their behavior with regard to eating and exercise habits.

9-36 The CDCP Guidelines do not endorse extracurricular physical activity programs in schools.

9-37 The CDCP Guidelines support daily physical education in grades K–12.

9-38 One criticism of the ACSM certification program is that many of the requirements are similar for the various levels, which, in essence, fails to discriminate between the various professions.

9-39 The YMCA's Healthy Back program is not another level of certification but rather an additional course of study available for people who have passed the basic fitness leader level.

9-40 Sports participation increases from ages 10 to 14.

9-41 Lack of appropriate physical activity patterns among youth is considered by most to be a national problem.

9-42 Evidence suggests that exercise involvement decreases throughout adulthood and then increases in the senior years.

True-False Answers

1. T	7. F	13. T	19. T	25. F	31. F	37. T
2. T	8. T	14. T	20. F	26. F	32. F	38. F
3. F	9. T	15. T	21. T	27. F	33. T	39. T
4. T	10. T	16. F	22. T	28. F	34. T	40. F
5. F	11. T	17. T	23. T	29. T	35. T	41. T
6. F	12. F	18. F	24. T	30. T	36. F	42. T

Short Answer Questions

9-1 What are the five major factors athletic and fitness administrators feel contribute to a growing interest in fitness facilities?

ans: a. Media portrays a "fit" image
           b. Income available for recreation
           c. Women's movement; fitness for women is acceptable
           d. Influence of the Olympic Games
           e. Greater emphasis by medical and health professions

9-2 What are the three reasons for increased corporate support of fitness programs?

ans: a. Increase worker productivity
           b. Decrease employee absenteeism
           c. Decrease medical costs

9-3 Identify the six levels of certification developed by the American College of Sports Medicine (ACSM).

ans: a. Program director
           b. Exercise specialist
           c. Exercise test technologist
           d. Health/fitness director
           e. Health/fitness instructor
           f. Exercise leader aerobics

9-4 What is the death rate from degenerative disease among persons who are physically active as compared to the death rate among those with an inactive lifestyle?

ans: The death rate of active persons is one-half that of inactive ones.

9-5 What are the normal methods for obtaining information about the activity lifestyle of people? Why are varied results often obtained?

ans: Questionnaires and interviews produce varied results because of definitions used and inaccurate self-reporting. Also, the fitness "boom" is a yuppie phenomenon. If this is the population surveyed, results will be different than if different socioeconomic classes are included.

9-6 Why are historical comparisons of children/youth fitness difficult to make?

ans: Fitness tests in the past have emphasized motor performance items rather than health fitness items.

9-7 What were the two areas for concern on the NCYFS I?

ans: a. High levels of body composition (skinfold test)
       b. Poor cardiovascular scores (mile run/walk)

9-8 Why has concern for children/youth fitness recently become more serious?

ans: Scientists and the medical community have now firmly established a link between children/youth health fitness and adult degenerative disease.

9-9 What are the main policy implications of the CDCP Guidelines?

ans: a. The physical activity needs of students must be addressed throughout the school.
       b. The school must link to the community and the home to fully address the physical activity needs of students.

9-10 What two activities can burn 2000 calories in three hours?

ans: Running and cross-country skiing

9-11 In general, what percentage of boys and girls participate on interscholastic sport teams?

ans: About 50–60% of boys and 38–43% of girls

9-12 Why are data on children's activity participation difficult to assess?

ans: Information is obtained from parents, who tend not to be reliable about their children's activity participation.

9-13 What kinds of fitness programs have been established in schools?

ans: a. Schoolwide programs at the elementary level
      b. Remediation programs
      c. Home based programs
      d. Fitness clubs
      e. Required and elective fitness courses

9-14 What problem exists with trying to implement fitness programs in physical education classes?

ans: Inadequate time allotment

9-15 How many children in the United States take physical education classes from a specialist?

ans: Fewer than half

9-16 What is the status of physical education requirements in the various states?

ans: In general, the requirements have been decreasing.

9-17 What two main components are required for worksite or employee fitness programs?

ans: a. Time
      b. Facilities

9-18 What are indicators of the size of the home fitness market?

ans: The amount of merchandise sold: shoes, videotapes, bicycles, home exercise equipment, etc.

9-19 Why is behavior change associated with fitness so difficult?

ans: Most health benefits are long term and are not good motivators. The benefits of knowledge about fitness need to be promoted so as to motivate people.

9-20 What historically has most often triggered the federal government's concern with fitness?

ans: High rates of draft rejections during wartime based on lack of fitness

9-21 Why was the President's Council on Youth Physical Fitness established?

ans: It was a response to the national concern that resulted when American children were shown to be considerably less fit than European children on the Kraus-Weber tests.

9-22 What has been the role of the federal government in the promotion of fitness?

ans: It has been supportive through the work of various committees and councils, but no monetary commitments have been made to date.

9-23 What is the CATCH program?

ans: The Child and Adolescent Trial for Cardiovascular Health—a school-based program involving PE, nutrition, and classroom instruction

9-24 What is a Fitnessgram?

ans: A computerized report card on a student's level of health-related fitness along with suggestions on how to improve the child's score sponsored by AAHPERD, the Institute for Aerobic Research, and the Campbell Soup Company

9-25 What licensing/certification is required to teach in a fitness program?

ans: None!

9-26 What is probably the single most important reason for supporting the continued development and expansion of school fitness programs?

ans: They are taught by certified physical education teachers who typically have had training in courses that are relevant to planning and implementing fitness programs.

9-27 What is the ACSM?

ans: The American College of Sports Medicine is a national organization of those interested in the investigation and implementation of good fitness programs.

9-28 Why does the ACSM have certification levels?

ans: To ensure that persons with ACSM certification have the necessary knowledge and experience to plan and implement appropriate fitness programs for clients

9-29 What are the major risk factors associated with cardiovascular disease?

ans: High blood pressure, high cholesterol, smoking, and inactivity

9-30 What projects has AAHPERD sponsored to help promote fitness?

ans: a. President's Council awards
       b. Fitnessgram
       c. Jump Rope for Heart
       d. Created a position for a Director of Fitness Projects
       e. Promoted research via convention programs, conferences, and publications
       f. Physical Best

Chapter 10

Problems and Issues in Fitness

Discussions in this chapter should focus on the *real* evidence of widespread lack of fitness among children and youth and the socioeconomic basis of fitness involvement among adults. Lifestyle problems can often be addressed by starting from where your students are in terms of a personal program of fitness. Developing "ideal" programs for specific contexts can also be an entry into discussions about alternative solutions.

True-False Questions

10-1 Fitness is important because many jobs in the modern era require a high level of fitness to perform well.

10-2 A major aim of fitness advocates is a more productive life rather than a longer life.

10-3 An important reason for improving the fitness of older citizens is the high level of health costs for this age group.

10-4 Fitness programs that aim at quick, large changes are likely to be the most effective because of their results.

10-5 If an individual keeps himself or herself fit, then the expenses attributed to an unhealthy population can be avoided by that person.

10-6 Persons who are most at-risk for health problems are those for whom fitness information is least accessible.

10-7 The aversive immediate consequences attributed to aerobic activity often govern the behavior of individuals instead of the long-term positive consequences of such activity.

10-8 The Corbin model suggests that once people start exercising and become fit, they will maintain fitness for the rest of their life.

10-9 Research shows that programs that develop a lifestyle emphasis tend to produce commitment for participants.

10-10 The thin, hard body portrayed by the media as a fit person gives an ideal standard to which all fitness-conscious adults should strive.

10-11 Celebrities who have taken an interest in fitness activities have done much to promote and exemplify scientific fitness training principles.

10-12 Although substantial fitness knowledge has been gained in the past several decades, extensive, current research activity promises to greatly increase this knowledge.

10-13 Straight-legged situps and bent knee situps with the hands behind the head have both been shown to be potentially dangerous exercises.

10-14 Fitness gains can be monitored by weighing in on accurate scales twice a week.

10-15 The major means of better educating the public about fitness will be through health and physical education programs in the schools.

10-16 The knowledge base required for certification by the American College of Sports Medicine (ACSM) and the YMCA is more extensive than that required by a physical education teacher.

10-17 Individuals who were used to establish fitness norms were required to pass basic fitness requirements before their results could be used for data.

10-18 An individual who scores at the 80th percentile on a fitness test would be considered to be highly fit whereas someone on the 50th percentile would be said to have only average fitness.

10-19 A teenage girl could alternate between a recreational jogging pace and a brisk walk and obtain an "average" score on the one-mile-run fitness test.

10-20 When standards are used for comparisons on fitness tests, students can tell how their scores relate to others in the population being tested.

10-21 As the percentage of Americans becoming senior citizens increases, health care costs as well as the quality of their lives will motivate people to seek out new physical education programs.

10-22 As Americans reach retirement, they have more time and tend to engage in appropriate fitness activities.

10-23 Physical educators in setting up programs for seniors must realize that persons "slow down" when they get older.

10-24 Dr. Kenneth Cooper, a leader in the fitness movement, feels that recent gains made against heart disease will be wiped out in the next twenty years because of poor fitness levels in children.

10-25 Cooper sees a major part of the problem of fitness to be a lack of commitment to physical fitness by parents of today's youth.

10-26 School-based fitness programs tend to emphasize fitness testing but fail to give prescriptive programs to improve fitness levels.

10-27 Corbin feels that many fitness programs consist of boring activities with inadequate challenge, which tend to turn students off to fitness.

10-28 A physical education teacher can implement a computerized fitness program called Fitnessgram that will assess current fitness levels of children.

10-29 Students must exercise five days per week in vigorous aerobic activity before a fitness benefit is realized.

10-30 Research has shown exercise to enhance the body's immune system response, thus making it more resistant to all disease.

10-31 Because of the lack of television and other financial and entertainment diversions, low income adults tend to be more fit than their above average income counterparts.

10-32 The primary purpose of fitness testing should be for diagnosis and feedback to individuals taking the test.

10-33 Good fitness programs in schools are probably the best available solution to the national problem of fitness.

10-34 Physical education teachers usually incorporate a fitness component in every class period.

10-35 A physical activity infrastructure includes facilities but not programs.

10-36 Since seniors tend to lose the competitive spirit, activities for this age group must be of a non-competitive nature.

10-37 Access to fitness information and facilities is strongly related to socioeconomic status.

10-38 The American Public Health Association has argued that fitness programs must be embedded in the community rather than in schools if they are to be effective.

True-False Answers

1. F	7. T	13. T	19. T	25. F	31. F	37. T
2. T	8. F	14. F	20. F	26. T	32. T	38. F
3. T	9. T	15. T	21. T	27. T	33. T	
4. F	10. F	16. F	22. F	28. T	34. F	
5. F	11. F	17. F	23. F	29. F	35. F	
6. T	12. T	18. F	24. T	30. F	36. F	

Short Answer Questions

10-1 What is the major fitness problem among physical education teachers?

ans: Time

10-2 What five steps does Corbin feel need to be incorporated into a fitness program?

ans: a. Do regular exercise
       b. Achieve physical fitness
       c. Develop personal exercise patterns
       d. Evaluate yourself
       e. Plan and use information to solve problems

10-3 List five reasons why school-based fitness programs do not succeed.

ans: a. Overemphasis on periodic testing with no follow up/prescriptive programming
       b. Boring fitness activities
       c. Inadequate challenge and incentive in fitness classes
       d. Too much reliance on regimentation
       e. Too little time to shower and dismal locker facilities

10-4 What equity issues are most prominent in fitness?

ans: a. Gender
       b. Race
       c. Socioeconomic status

10-5 What socioeconomic and age group has most been a part of the fitness boom?

ans: Young and above average income

10-6 What guidelines are suggested for fitness testing?

ans: a. Should identify at-risk children
       b. Award systems based on criterion-referenced standards
       c. Accumulated physical activity used as well as fitness performance
       d. Use self-testing
       e. Primary purpose of diagnosis and feedback related to goals

10-7 How do health care costs affect all Americans indirectly even though the person himself or herself may be physically fit?

ans: a. Health insurance costs are increasing
       b. As absenteeism rises, productivity goes down
       c. Public funds are utilized

10-8 Why do 90% of Americans believe exercise is good for them while few actually follow through and exercise on a regular basis?

ans: The consequences of regular involvement in appropriate aerobic activity are typically long term, while the immediate consequences are aversive to many people.

10-9 What must happen before a satisfactory solution to inadequate fitness is found?

ans: A change of lifestyle must occur. No "quick fix" fitness program will be sustained.

10-10 What three things must the average person know if the general public is to be considered "educated" about fitness?

ans: The average person will know about:

       a. The different kinds of fitness
       b. What needs to be done to develop and maintain health fitness
       c. The fitness products and services that are appropriate to fitness goals

10-11 In what three ways do the media create problems with educating the general public about fitness?

ans: a. The body associated with "fitness" is not necessary for health fitness, nor is it obtainable for most people.
       b. The impression is given that fitness miracles can occur immediately and with little effort.
       c. The celebrities who represent fitness know little specific information about fitness and often convey misinformation.

10-12 What are some examples of public misinformation about fitness?

ans: a. Professionals and exercise leaders are doing exercises that have been shown to
           be potentially dangerous even though a safer substitute exists.
        b. People are weight conscious, not fat conscious, and subsequently get
           frustrated by not having a weight loss after they begin an exercise program.

10-13 What will probably be the source for educating the public about fitness?

ans: The schools

10-14 What requirements are necessary for many of the aerobic fitness certificates?

ans: Most requirements, if any, are minimal. In some instances certification can be
obtained by mail order.

10-15 Why should standards for fitness replace the current system of norms?

ans: The norms give a relationship to other children. Since American children are
basically unfit, comparisons are made to a less than desirable number. If standards were
used, students would be encouraged to work toward achieving a score that would
represent an appropriate level of fitness.

10-16 What are the economic and social consequences that encourage seniors to be fit?

ans: a. Economic: high costs for health care for seniors
        b. Social: increase the quality of life for senior citizens

10-17 What are three reasons that stand in the way for older adults to participate in health
fitness programs?

ans: a. They have excessive fears about participating in activities
        b. They underestimate their physical capabilities
        c. They overestimate the value of the light, infrequent activity in which they
           engage

10-18 What seems to be more appropriate than the traditional myth that persons "slow
down" because they get older?

ans: Persons get older because they slow down.

10-19 How could seniors be better educated about lifetime fitness and a physically active lifestyle?

ans:　　a.　Better information among seniors about physical fitness in old age
　　　　b.　More programs that involve appropriate levels of aerobic activity
　　　　c.　More publicity for senior role models so that others can be encouraged to exercise and compete vigorously

10-20 According to Cooper, what factor could possibly negate all of the gains made against heart disease over the past twenty years?

ans: The low level of fitness among children

10-21 What two characteristics are true of the majority of people in the fitness boom?

ans:　　a.　Young
　　　　b.　Above average income

10-22 Discuss briefly the problems associated with fitness.

ans:　　a.　Certification of fitness instructor/leaders
　　　　b.　Inadequate definition of/role model for fitness by the general public
　　　　c.　The norms used for comparison are inadequate

10-23 What is referred to when citing the structural problems of fitness and fitness education?

ans: The fact that access to fitness information, nutritious food at reasonable prices, and fitness facilities is less likely for lower socioeconomic groups.

Chapter 11

Basic Concepts of Physical Education

Try having students articulate their own philosophy of physical education before reading this chapter, then compare and contrast their philosophies with what they read. Have students respond to the models. Which sound like the most fun for students? Which sound like the best to teach? Which best reflect the students' own philosophy? How do the models compare with what they experienced in school? A good way to close is to have students discuss and agree on class goals for physical education.

True-False Questions

11-1 Although physical education programs look quite different from school to school, there is widespread agreement on the basic definition of physical education.

11-2 The most important model for physical education in this century has been the developmental model.

11-3 A major tenet of the progressive education movement was the cognitive development of young people, which explains the emphasis on academic testing in physical education.

11-4 Sport had been advocated as part of the physical education curriculum even as early as the Boston Conference in 1889.

11-5 Clark Hetherington has been called the Father of Modern Physical Education largely because of his succinct statement of the "education through the physical" viewpoint.

11-6 The multi-activity program was first established in the eclectic curriculum.

11-7 "Education through the physical" fit completely with the goals of progressive education.

11-8 The motor development objective dealt with what is now called the health fitness component.

11-9 Group activities are often incorporated into physical education lesson plans to meet the social development objective.

11-10 With the increased importance of sport, the multi-activity approach used a variety of sports, both individual and team, but excluded the gymnastics and dance that had been the basis of early physical education.

11-11 The multi-activity approach offered various sports for extended periods of time, kept students on a single team, and created a final championship event that allowed students to experience many of the benefits that belonging to a team can bring.

11-12 The PEPI program represented a radical departure from the "education through the physical" program.

11-13 Sport units are commonly incorporated in movement education, but concepts such as striking and force absorption are emphasized rather than rules and competitive games.

11-14 Problem solving, guided discovery, and movement exploration are teaching styles utilized in movement education.

11-15 A final goal of movement education is not so much the actual movement but the ability of the students to make good movement decisions that would contribute to an independence even after the completion of education.

11-16 Competition is downplayed in movement education while creativity and aesthetics are stressed.

11-17 Movement education has been most popular in high school settings where students choose electives for their physical education curriculum.

11-18 The Health-Related Physical Education approach to physical education attempts to teach students to maintain a healthy lifestyle and to be knowledgeable consumers of fitness.

11-19 The humanistic education movement focuses attention on academic achievement and has been implemented in physical education, stressing strategies and the cognitive part of sport.

11-20 The social development model has been primarily used with troubled adolescent students, teaching first self-control and progressing at later stages to caring about others and leadership skills.

11-21 The NASPE outcomes for physical education are likely to be the dominant force in curriculum development in the foreseeable future.

11-22 The Basic Stuff series sought to integrate disciplinary knowledge into the regular physical education curriculum.

11-23 Sport education refers to the quality experiences students receive in the interscholastic sports programs in schools.

11-24 The sport education model is designed to teach not only a sport but also the lessons that come from team affiliations and end of the season tournaments.

11-25 In the sport education model, students can learn the role of participant, coach, referee, and administrator.

11-26 The idea that adventure activities involve risk has stymied the growth of such areas in physical education because of the negative impacts on young children and youth.

11-27 A goal of adventure education is for the student to gain enough skill to participate in the activity safely.

11-28 Adventure education seeks constantly to eliminate risk because anxiety will not allow the child to think clearly and may result in physical harm.

11-29 Administrators tend to discourage adventure education programs as the travel to the site takes time away from academic pursuits as well as costing the district more than the end results justify.

11-30 An eclectic model can include adventure, multi-activity, or social development models, the difference being that all courses are elective.

11-31 Schools are governed at the state rather than the federal level.

11-32 Laws supporting physical education at the elementary level are typically weak, allowing recess in some states to meet physical education requirements.

11-33 Most children in the United States do have physical education instruction from a physical education specialist, although not on a daily basis.

11-34 More than one-half of the states either have no high school physical education requirement or require only one semester or year for graduation.

11-35 Although increased physical education requirements have had support on the federal level, the state legislatures must pass laws before change will occur.

11-36 Liability and safety issues have virtually eliminated trampolines from public schools.

11-37 Because rappeling and rock climbing are relatively safe when done properly, they are incorporated into programs despite liability concerns.

11-38 Although athletics have a history of discrimination against females, physical education has not been plagued by these concerns.

11-39 The concept of inclusion suggests that all students with disabilities should be mainstreamed into regular physical education classes.

11-40 When one considers the "education through the physical" model, the activities themselves are not so important as what they accomplish for the students.

11-41 Title IX has ensured that there are as many female physical education teachers in high schools as there are male physical education teachers.

True-False Answers

1. F	7. T	13. F	19. F	25. T	31. T	37. T
2. T	8. F	14. T	20. T	26. F	32. T	38. F
3. F	9. T	15. T	21. T	27. T	33. F	39. T
4. F	10. T	16. T	22. T	28. F	34. T	40. T
5. T	11. F	17. F	23. F	29. F	35. T	41. F
6. F	12. F	18. T	24. T	30. F	36. T	

Short Answer Questions

11-1 What were the four phases of education that Hetherington thought to be the scope of the *new* physical education?

ans: a. Organic education
        b. Psychomotor education
        c. Character education
        d. Intellectual education

11-2 What is a developmental model that uses individual and team sports, dance, gymnastics, fitness, and adventure activities for the physical education program and presents these in blocks or units?

ans: Multi-activity program

11-3 What is the PEPI program?

ans: A public information program sponsored by AAHPERD designed to enhance the image of physical education and to inform the public about these goals

11-4 What were the five areas of concern for the PEPI program?

ans: a. Physical and motor skill
        b. Health
        c. Academic achievement
        d. Positive self-concept
        e. Social skills

11-5 What are the three main purposes of movement education?

ans: a. Skillful, versatile, effective, and efficient movement in situations requiring
            planned or unplanned responses
        b. Awareness of the meaning, significance, feeling, and joy of movement both
            as a performer and as an observer
        c. Acquisition and application of the knowledge that governs human movement

11-6 What are the two sets of goals in the Adventure Education model?

ans: a. To gain skill, participate safely, and gain satisfaction from participation
        b. To teach problem-solving techniques, enhance self-concept, and increase
            personal growth

11-7 What are the five defining characteristics of sport education?

ans: a. Typically done in seasons
        b. Players affiliate with a single team for the season
        c. A formal competition is arranged
        d. A culminating event determines the winner of the competition
        e. Records are kept and published to enhance and build interest

11-8 What skills are required of an adventure education teacher?

ans: Teachers must have skills to interact with and guide students during the travel to the
site as well as in risky situations. Also, the teacher should have substantial experience
with the skills/activity being taught.

11-9 What current area of emphasis reflects physical education's early background in
medicine?

ans: Fitness

11-10 Why was the progressive education movement important to contemporary physical education?

ans: Through progressive education, physical education came to be considered as a valuable school subject.

11-11 What major tenet of progressive education recognized the importance of physical education?

ans: The tenet was that all education should contribute to the development of the *whole* child.

11-12 What physical education philosophy was a direct result of the developmental perspective of progressive education?

ans: "Education through the physical"

11-13 Why was sport incorporated into physical education curriculums?

ans: Students loved sport and wanted to have the opportunity to participate in sport while in school, despite the wishes of school and university.

11-14 What term is used for the physical education developmental model?

ans: "Education through the physical"

11-15 In which grade levels is movement education usually found?

ans: Elementary grades

11-16 What physical education philosophy was consistent with the goals of progressive education?

ans: "Education through the physical"

11-17 How might Heatherington's four objectives be reflected in the parts of a physical education lesson plan today?

ans: Opening calisthenics are included for meeting the fitness objective. Skills drills are organized to meet the motor development objective. Tests on rules address the mental development. Group activities are used to promote social development.

11-18 What rationale was behind the multi-activity program?

ans: In order to ensure the *full* development of the child or youth, a variety of activities were planned for the students.

11-19 What monograph came as close to a national curriculum for physical education as we have ever come? What committee produced this and who was the chair?

ans: The Physical Education Curriculum, prepared in 1927 by a committee sponsored by the College Physical Education Association and chaired by William Ralph La Porte

11-20 How does the organization of human movement units differ from that of sport or fitness units?

ans: The units are defined by movement concepts instead of sport activities. Striking or absorbing force might be units instead of basketball, as in a sports unit, or strength, as in a fitness unit.

11-21 What five concepts are emphasized with a movement education teaching style?

ans: a. Problem solving
        b. Guided discovery
        c. Exploration
        d. Acceptance
        e. Success

11-22 As competition is minimized in movement education, what other aspect of movement is emphasized?

ans: The aesthetic dimension, as teachers tend to stress creativity and aesthetic enjoyment over objective performance

11-23 What two goals are stressed in the Health Related Physical Education model?

ans: a. Contributes to the amount of moderate to intense physical activity students get in physical education
        b. Influences them to lead more physically active lives outside of physical education class

11-24 What three types of activities are usually found in movement education curriculums?

ans: a. Educational gymnastics
        b. Educational dance
        c. Educational games

11-25 What is the major advantage of HRPE?

ans: There have been several well funded program trials of various kinds throughout the United States.

11-26 What is the purpose of integration in the Academic-Integration model?

ans: To achieve synthesis between traditionally diverse forms of knowledge

11-27 Differentiate between internal and external integration.

ans: Internal: physical education provides a curriculum model for other disciplines to
              adopt
          External: physical education is integrated with other classroom subjects

11-28 What series of booklets that focuses on a disciplinary concept curriculum has recently been published by AAHPERD?

ans: *Basic Stuff*

11-29 What are the two integrating goals of the many diverse models that together constituted humanistic education?

ans: a. Treating students as individuals
          b. Focusing on personal growth and social development rather than academic
              achievement

11-30 From what curriculum philosophy and concept did the sport education model develop?

ans: Play education and the concept of play

11-31 On what type of student has the social development model been used most often?

ans: The troubled adolescent student

11-32 What type of teacher is required for a social development program?

ans: One who is authentic and caring. One who can tolerate student differences and be secure and firm enough to deal with them.

11-33 What is the content of the sport education model?

ans: Physical education as sport

11-34 What assumption does the sport education model make about *good* competition?

ans: It is fun and educationally useful.

11-35 How are daily lessons spent in a sport education model?

ans: Daily lessons consist of practice and competition with more time devoted to competition as the season progresses.

11-36 What is the teacher's role in a sport education model?

ans: The teacher is very much like a coach, although the model calls for student coaches to assume major responsibility for their teams.

11-37 What two trends have led to the adventure education curriculum?

ans: a. The idea that adventure activities had potential for education and character development
     b. Substantial increase in public interest in outdoor recreation

11-38 Why is risk frequently included in adventure education?

ans: The assumption is that risk produces anxiety and stress for the participant. The participant learns to deal with the stress and to overcome the anxiety. Since this is often done with a group, interaction with group members also becomes an educational focus.

11-39 Why doesn't offering a great variety of courses in an eclectic curriculum necessarily mean the program is a good one?

ans: Quantity should not be confused with quality.

11-40 What is the negative side of liability?

ans: Activities are not done for fear of liability. Teachers are discouraged from being innovative with equipment.

11-41 What has been the trend for physical education requirements at the state level?

ans: Mandatory time has decreased. In some situations the laws about elementary physical education are so weak, recess has been used to fulfill physical education requirements. Fewer than half the children in the United States get physical education from a specialist, and many of those who do only see a specialist once or twice a week.

11-42 What is the positive side of liability in physical education?

ans: Teachers plan activities more carefully, check equipment more often, supervise more closely, and make sure that students are ready for the activity.

11-43 Why did Title IX affect physical education and athletics in most schools?

ans: It affected any educational program receiving federal funding. Since most schools receive some form of federal assistance, physical education and sport were included under its jurisdiction.

11-44 What are four changes that have occurred in physical education as a direct result of Title IX?

ans: a. Coeducational classes
         b. Assignment of teachers based on skill rather than gender
         c. Grouping on ability rather than gender
         d. Equal access for boys and girls to the entire physical education curriculum

11-45 What was the main feature of Public Law 94-142?

ans: To ensure that all disabled children receive a free, appropriate public education, which includes all services necessary to meet their unique needs

11-46 What does the term "mainstreaming" mean in relation to physical education?

ans: Disabled students are put into a regular physical education class instead of being separated into special classes composed of disabled students.

11-47 What is more important in the "education through the physical" model than the activities themselves?

ans: What the activities are used to accomplish

Chapter 12

Physical Education Programs and Professions

This is another chapter that is good to "localize." How do area programs compare to the models described? How close is quality, daily physical education in area schools? What are requirements in your state? What schools go beyond them? A discussion of the roles played by physical educators is often enlivened by references to physical educators experienced during the students' K–12 years.

True-False Questions

12-1 Curricular models such as adventure education and movement education are only found in public school settings.

12-2 Students don't get as much time in physical education throughout their schooling as a high school varsity athlete would get in interscholastic sports.

12-3 The minimum requirements for education are specified by Federal Title acts.

12-4 Even though physical education is required at the elementary level in more than 75% of the states, requirements are so loosely written that many programs use recess to satisfy them.

12-5 Realizing the importance of fitness in adulthood, the trend has been to increase requirements in physical education for high school graduation.

12-6 Because wealthier people belong to health and country clubs, physical education requirements in their districts tend to be less than for less affluent districts.

12-7 Trends over the past twenty-five years indicate that state requirements for physical education are getting weaker rather than stronger.

12-8 Physical education must be defined by what takes place, the goals that are being pursued, and the setting in which this all occurs.

12-9 Exemplary programs usually need extra effort and leadership from either individual teachers or departments to be both started and maintained.

12-10 Teachers who have coaching responsibilities usually have mediocre physical education classes.

12-11 Although one does not have to be a certified teacher to teach for a "Y" or recreation center, such certification does give one an edge when applying for jobs.

12-12 Sport education is not an appropriate model for the elementary school.

12-13 Most school districts use curriculum planners or buy a curriculum package rather than having district teachers write their own curriculum.

12-14 Since schools have a trained counseling staff, most physical education teachers choose to send students to this department rather than talking with students themselves.

12-15 Standards for teachers are a major aspect of recent educational reform.

12-16 In recent years, most states require certification in a single subject area, whereas in the past teachers were required to have a teaching major and one or two minors, all of which they could teach.

12-17 To develop a fitness-emphasis program for high school students would be to narrow the physical education program too much.

12-18 Although certification varies from state to state, the basic field of study for physical education majors is consistent across the United States.

12-19 Movement education programs seem to be confined primarily to the early elementary grades.

12-20 NASPE Standards for beginning teachers suggest a series of dispositions that are the basis for professional practice.

12-21 The Individuals with Disabilities Act (IDEA) clearly lists required qualifications for personnel to work with students with disabilities.

True-False Answers

1. F	6. F	11. T	16. F	21. F
2. T	7. T	12. F	17. F	
3. F	8. F	13. F	18. F	
4. T	9. T	14. F	19. T	
5. F	10. F	15. T	20. T	

Short Answer Questions

12-1 What are four things exemplary programs have in common?

ans: a. Leadership has been exerted by physical educator(s) to get the program started and to maintain it.
b. Each program stands for something specific.
c. Programs are exciting for students.
d. Teachers responsible for these programs did not have major coaching responsibilities.

12-2 What are the three levels of certification available for physical education teachers?

ans: a. K–6
b. 7–12
c. K–12

12-3 Give some examples of how technology is being used in physical education.

ans: a. Heartrate monitors to track exercise patterns
b. Use of the internet to take part in newsgroups related to physical activity
c. Student teachers use video records to analyze and improve their teaching.

12-4 A home-based activity program is a component of which model?

ans: Comprehensive Health Related Elementary School Model

12-5 How are minimum requirements for education determined?

ans: They are typically specified by state law.

12-6 When states require physical education but fail to specify time or activity guidelines, what is the result?

ans: Schools can do virtually anything they want to in order to meet the requirement and can count such things as recess, class play time, etc.

12-7 At what age level is there the largest physical education requirement, including specific time/unit specification?

ans: Grades 7, 8, and 9

12-8 What are the optimistic and pessimistic outlooks about minimum state requirements for physical education?

ans: Optimistic: Most school districts go beyond minimum requirements and hire specialists
        Pessimistic: State requirements are written so loosely that they can be ignored

12-9 What has been the trend for physical education state requirements over the past twenty-five years?

ans: The requirements have gotten weaker rather than stronger.

12-10 What community agencies can be linked with a high school physical education program to add interesting and challenging activities to the curriculum?

ans: Local fire department, Parks and Recreation Department, U.S. Tennis Association, Pro Golfers Association-First Swing Program, U. S. Rowing

12-11 What are some ways physical education teachers use computers in their daily work?

ans: a. Word processing
        b. Database management for attendance and grades
        c. Assessment of fitness and motor skills

12-12 What are some ways physical education teachers can continue their professional development?

ans: Through journals, conferences, staff development programs, and professional contacts at other schools and in the community

12-13 What are the expectations when teachers represent their school, the physical education profession, and the teaching profession in general?

ans: They are expected to be knowledgeable and to behave in a professional manner.

12-14 Who makes rules for teacher certification?

ans: State legislatures

12-15 Why do some states require teaching minors?

ans: In states with smaller schools, principals will be able to utilize staff more effectively if teachers are able to teach more than one subject area.

12-16 What are field- or school-based experiences? Give examples.

ans: There are situations where the teacher candidate is in a school working with students. These can range from observation to full-scale teaching as is done in a student teaching experience.

12-17 What are some of the non-teaching roles of a physical educator?

ans: a. Planner
      b. Manager
      c. Colleague
      d. Professional physical educator
      e. Counselor
      f. Representative of the school

12-18 Describe each of the three ways teacher certification can vary from state to state.

ans: a. Level of certification
      b. Number of teaching specialties
      c. Amount of field experience

Chapter 13

Problems and Issues in Physical Education

This is a good opportunity for small group work—each group taking a problem, discussing, and reporting solutions to the class. If you discussed goals in Chapter 11, this is a good point to use them to define the subject matter called physical education. Another good discussion issue is to define the content of a national curriculum, as if one were going to be instituted. Equity issues deserve careful attention and discussion.

True-False Questions

13-1 Because habits of participation develop during childhood, unfit children tend to remain so through adolescence and adulthood.

13-2 Recess is not considered by schools to be "physical education time."

13-3 Surveys done in physical education tend not to give a true picture of actual practice, as respondents report what should be done according to district rules rather than according to actual practice.

13-4 The back to basics movement has helped increase physical education time at the elementary level.

13-5 Although state laws do not specify that a specialist teacher has to provide physical education instruction, a recent survey indicated that the vast majority of children in grades 1–4 have a physical education teacher.

13-6 Most classroom teachers have a good preparation in physical education and seem eager to provide instruction on the days when the physical education teacher is not scheduled to meet with their classes.

13-7 Some physical education specialists provide instruction at several schools during the course of one week.

13-8 COPECs developmentally appropriate practices document provides a thorough checklist of specific practices that should be avoided in elementary physical education.

13-9 In a good physical education program with a quality instructor, facilities will not affect what is being taught.

13-10 Most professionals generally agree that a skill-oriented curriculum is the most beneficial for elementary students.

13-11 Most elementary education specialists use the national curriculum advocated by AAHPERD rather than writing their own.

13-12 High school physical education has been described as an endangered species, which means that it might become extinct if it continues on its present course.

13-13 Research shows that many high school physical educators judge the success of their program by whether or not they keep their students busy, happy, and good.

13-14 Physical education programs that amount to being a supervised recreation program occur when administrators and teachers have low expectations.

13-15 Many who have assessed the problems of secondary physical education agree that the multi-activity curriculum contributes to a general lack of outcomes.

13-16 A smorgasbord approach of giving a variety of sports, dance, etc. activities is generally thought to be the best approach to a high school curriculum.

13-17 While the amount of time spent in elementary physical education has stayed the same, the time required at the secondary level has been increased by most states.

13-18 To better serve high school students, most school districts support an elective physical education program that exceeds state requirements.

13-19 When physical education classes are overcrowded, problems with class management, equipment, and space can arise.

13-20 Schools that have elective classes or programs based upon skill progression greatly reduce the problem of skill heterogeneity.

13-21 In some ways, problems associated with co-ed physical education classes are actually problems related to heterogeneity of skills.

13-22 Role conflict can occur when teaching and coaching require more time or energy than the person has to give.

13-23 Teaching tends to offer many types of social reinforcement whereas coaching often causes a person to work long hours without social reinforcement.

13-24 To solve the teacher/coach role conflict, some have suggested giving teachers a lighter schedule during their sport season(s).

13-25 Most school districts have full-scale intramural programs so as to accommodate athletes eliminated in the varsity sports model.

13-26 Western education philosophies see the mind and body as separate entities and often choose to educate the mind rather than the body and mind as an integrated whole.

13-27 Many parents do not support physical education because of their own negative experience with the subject when they were in school.

13-28 Students must be able to identify areas of improvement (fitness, skill, knowledge) that have been the direct result of a physical education class if it is to be a viable part of a school curriculum.

13-29 Although communication of physical education outcomes to parents and students is important, this needs to be preceded by a statement of purpose if a program is going to be effective.

13-30 Before problems of class size, poor facilities, and non-support from administrators will be changed, a quality physical education program must be built.

13-31 The national curriculum written by AAHPERD grew out of the lack of understanding of what physical education should be and what students need to achieve it.

13-32 Some experts have argued that secondary physical education is in such trouble that it needs to be replaced, not repaired.

13-33 Liability issues have helped physical education in many ways in that teachers now are better supervisors of activities and give proper lead-ups for advanced skills.

13-34 If a teacher takes proper precautions to safeguard students from harm, courts probably would consider that the teacher had acted in a reasonable and prudent manner and not hold him/her liable.

13-35 Physical education has historically been a place where girls and women could be active and competitive, unlike other aspects of our society.

13-36 Since Title IX, research evidence suggests that girls get equal opportunities to boys in physical education.

13-37 Some physical educators have advocated that all competition is harmful (negative) for children.

13-38 When competition teaches students to use the rules to gain an advantage and the only way to win is to have the best score, it should be eliminated.

13-39 School physical education should provide the foundation from which community and private sector physical education grows and prospers.

13-40 School physical education has been directly responsible for the "fitness boom" and has become even more important in schools with the increased importance of fitness to adults.

True-False Answers

1. T	7. T	13. T	19. T	25. F	31. F	37. T
2. F	8. F	14. T	20. T	26. T	32. T	38. T
3. T	9. F	15. T	21. T	27. T	33. T	39. T
4. F	10. F	16. F	22. T	28. T	34. T	40. F
5. T	11. F	17. F	23. F	29. T	35. F	
6. F	12. T	18. F	24. T	30. T	36. F	

Short Answer Questions

13-1 What are two reasons why surveys have not given an accurate picture of physical education at the elementary level?

ans: a. Recess is counted as physical education time.
        b. People report what should be done according to the rules rather than what is actually done.

13-2 What are two problems a traveling specialist experiences?

ans: a. Lack of continuity
        b. Does not "belong" to any faculty

13-3 What conditions contribute to difficult teaching situations at the secondary level?

ans: a. Class size
        b. Heterogeneity of skill levels
        c. Co-ed teaching

13-4 What is meant by the term "role conflict"?

ans: When a physical education teacher also coaches, and the two schedules create stress and strain. The person doesn't know how to divide his/her energies and cannot do both effectively. The expectations for each are strongly incompatible.

13-5 What is meant by the phrase "dualistic traditions" when talking about Western educational philosophies?

ans: The mind is separated from the body with education of the whole person neglected in favor of subjects that affect mental functioning.

13-6 What does the evidence suggest will happen if children become obese, unfit, and non-active in childhood?

ans: They will remain so throughout their adolescence and adulthood.

13-7 How have dualistic traditions from Western cultures slowed the acceptance of physical education as an important school subject?

ans: Because the mind is separate from the body, Western education seeks to educate each separately rather than integrating the two. When budget constraints force a choice, physical education is sacrificed.

13-8 For most elementary physical educators, why is the biggest obstacle for accomplishing the goals of quality physical education said to be lack of time?

ans: For fitness goals alone to be achieved, children need to be involved in vigorous activity at least three times per week for a twenty-minute duration. This does not include other skill and movement lessons also associated with elementary physical education. A high percentage of children have physical education only once or twice a week, for typically a thirty-minute lesson, which clearly is not even enough time to accomplish fitness objectives.

13-9 How have many principals increased the amount of time spent on basic subjects?

ans: They have done so by reducing the time devoted to physical education, art, and music, none of which are considered basic in current educational reform.

13-10 What kind of physical education methods preparation is required of most elementary classroom teachers?

ans: Usually only one class

13-11 Why do children usually benefit from having a specialist teach physical education rather than a classroom teacher?

ans: a. Specialist teachers have more/better preparation in the subject areas.
         b. Classroom teachers have many other subjects for which to plan, and physical education is typically slighted.

13-12 In what way do teaching facilities affect the quality of the elementary physical education program?

ans: A fully equipped gymnasium will affect the choice of activities in physical education as well as the method by which they are taught. For example, if a teacher has lots of equipment there can be far less standing by students waiting to participate and more time spent in activity.

13-13 What is the debate between movement education specialists and traditionalists?

ans: Movement educators see traditional elementary physical education curriculums as too competitive, too oriented toward specific skill development, lacking in creativity, and potentially damaging to the child's self-concept. The traditionalist sees movement education as too fluffy, not leading to anything, difficult to teach, and with no clear outcomes.

13-14 Why has secondary physical education been described as an endangered species?

ans: If it continues on its present course, it will eventually not exist in the future.

13-15 What were the main criteria by which physical educators judged their own success?

ans: a. If students were kept involved in the activity (busy)
        b. If students enjoyed the class (happy)
        c. If students behaved well (good)

13-16 What is seen to be the main problem in secondary physical education?

ans: Lack of expectations for real learning outcomes

13-17 What criticism is connected with the typical multi-activity curriculum?

ans: a. It contributes to a general lack of outcomes.
        b. Short units provide insufficient depth to learning.
        c. Improvement, achievement, and mastery are themes not readily apparent.

13-18 What is necessary to help to focus a high school curriculum?

ans: Adopt a main theme for the curriculum

13-19 What makes increasing the amount of physical education difficult?

ans: a. State requirements for physical education are decreasing.
        b. Tax dollars are spent in other ways.

13-20 What problems are created when physical education classes are too large?

ans: Problems with classroom management, equipment, and space

13-21 Why does heterogeneity of skills present problems to a physical education teacher?

ans: Accommodating huge differences in skill levels is difficult. People at different skill levels will have different needs within the same sport.

13-22 How can difficulties in teaching co-educational physical education be reduced substantially?

ans: Plan programs and schedule events in ways that help to group students (male and female) of like interests and abilities together in physical education.

13-23 Why does the coaching role in role conflict frequently receive more attention?

ans: Coaching tends to receive more social reinforcement, whereas teaching tends to be more private.

13-24 Diagram a traditional pyramid model for a physical education program. Which has the least and most participation?

ans: Physical education has the most participation while sport has the least. Diagrammatically it would resemble a pyramid.

sport

intramurals

physical education

13-25 What are intramurals?

ans: An intramural program provides activity opportunities for those who are interested in extending their skills and engaging in more competitive situations. They are competitions in various sports between students within one school.

13-26 Why are intramurals not found in all schools?

ans: a. Lack of resources: there are inadequate funds to pay for them.
        b. Teachers have full loads and do not wish to have an additional assignment.
        c. Facilities are used by sports teams after school.
        d. Students don't want to go home and then return for intramurals.

13-27 What suggests that intramurals would be popular if available in schools?

ans: a. The popularity of intramurals in colleges and universities
        b. The strong success of community recreation programs

13-28 Why has physical education had to fight for its existence?

ans: Because it is seldom seen as being basic to the school curriculum

13-29 What would probably happen if physical education teachers would begin teaching toward goals and outcomes?

ans: A greater credibility among the lay public and education profession might be achieved. It is probably the first step to be taken before physical education will become better established in the curriculum.

13-30 What do proponents of a national physical education curriculum feel it will provide?

ans: A common foundation for skill knowledge and fitness

13-31 Why do people oppose a national physical education curriculum?

ans: a. Many fear a national curriculum would fail to consider local needs and interests.
        b. Creativity, leading to new valuable program ideas, would be stifled.
        c. Others fear that the curriculum would include only sports and games since that has been the dominant curricular approach in recent times.

13-32 How can a physical education teacher circumvent liability problems?

ans: Teachers need to be aware of the risks involved and take proper precautions to safeguard students from them. If precautions are taken, then teachers have acted as reasonable, prudent persons, and chances of liability are minimized.

13-33 Why was Title IX so badly needed in physical education and sport?

ans: Physical education and sport had long histories of inequity toward girls' and women's participation.

13-34 In what respects have liability concerns helped and hurt physical education?

ans: a. Teachers pay more attention to teaching procedures.
          b. Activities are planned more carefully and closer to the curriculum syllabus.
          c. Safety considerations are made when designing instruction.
          d. Skill progressions are utilized.
In a negative sense, teachers do not choose certain activities because of perceived liability risks.

13-35 What is meant by good and bad competition?

ans: Good competition creates a festival atmosphere, creates a forum within which children can benefit, involves rivalry and striving to do the best one can within the rules and traditions. Bad competition is that which assumes the only way to win is to have the best score and uses the rules to gain an advantage, ignoring the traditions and rivalries.

13-36 Why are community and private sector programs not the answer to children's sport participation?

ans: Unlike a school program, they do not reach all children.

13-37 What must happen if lifespan sport, fitness, and physical education are to become more of a reality in the future?

ans: School physical education must begin to achieve its goals more completely.

13-38 Why do physical educators in urban schools typically adopt social goals as their main curricular outcomes?

ans: Those social goals are primarily aimed at current behavior in class so that some semblance of order is maintained and confrontations among students and between students and teachers is less likely.

Chapter 14

Exercise Physiology

Visits to labs or sports medicine clinics are helpful. Having the class watch a treadmill test or underwater weighing brings the specialization closer to the students' experiences. It is good to examine area universities where specializations exist—prerequisites, requirements, job opportunities.

True-False Questions

14-1 The scientific traditions of physical education were the measurement and promotion of fitness.

14-2 Because of its technical nature, language and terminology used by exercise physiologists remain beyond the understanding of most laypersons.

14-3 In the not too recent past, coaches did not allow athletes to drink water during practices and games, as they wanted to "toughen up" the players.

14-4 Because of the research in exercise physiology, swimmers have learned that lifting weights is detrimental to their optimal performances.

14-5 Exercise physiologists are trying to answer questions about optimal work and rest time periods for interval training.

14-6 Oxygen utilization research is for exercises that last longer than one minute.

14-7 Exercise metabolism concerns itself with how oxygen is utilized in the cardiovascular system.

14-8 Cardiac rehabilitation involves prescriptive work in preventing cardiovascular trauma as well as rehabilitating persons who have experienced cardiac problems.

14-9 Exercise biochemistry has become a major clinical extension of exercise physiology.

14-10 Exercise physiology is committed to health and fitness but does not work with improving motor performance.

14-11 Strength training would be considered an extension of the field of exercise physiology.

14-12 George Gerber, who came to be called the Father of Exercise Physiology, began speaking out about some of the claims that could not be substantiated by research.

14-13 By the 1920s muscle and exercise physiology had developed to the point that it was considered quite different from physiology and biochemistry.

14-14 Research money has been scarce for exercise physiology, which is why those scientists have stayed with physical education and athletics—to utilize the budgets of those departments.

14-15 Exercise physiology is probably the most popular and well-known physical education subdiscipline.

14-16 Spot reducing does appear to be effective in trimming fat, especially for the thigh and buttocks areas.

14-17 Weight can be lost through heat, but this is temporary rather than permanent.

14-18 A popular myth is that running farther rather than faster is the better approach to cardiovascular fitness.

14-19 The extraordinary increase in the sale of home exercise equipment could be viewed as one example of the interest in the areas studied by exercise physiologists.

14-20 With the purchase of home exercise equipment, physical education teachers are finally beginning to see that interest in adult fitness is extending to children and youth.

14-21 A clinical exercise physiologist might study the effects of exercise on diabetes, coronary heart disease, and cancer.

14-22 The age that fitness training should be introduced to children would be a topic studied by a clinical exercise physiologist.

14-23 Exercise physiologists might be found in departments of sport sciences, physical education, and veterinary medicine.

14-24 The primary function of a clinical exercise physiologist is to work with post-cardiac patients.

14-25 A small college department would probably elect to focus on exercise biochemistry, as that line of research is the least expensive.

14-26 Athletic training professionals would not be considered as belonging under the exercise physiology umbrella.

14-27 Adult fitness professionals are hired to work in employee fitness programs to improve fitness of employees and reduce insurance costs.

14-28 A typical undergraduate physical education major, with a teacher preparation emphasis, does not have the prerequisites necessary for a graduate program in exercise physiology.

14-29 A masters degree program in exercise physiology would prepare a person to work in a cardiac rehabilitation program.

14-30 A basic exercise physiology researcher tries to answer questions of an immediate applied nature.

14-31 Exercise physiology has become so successful that it has increasingly moved away from the field of sport.

14-32 Money to support research in exercise science comes from athletic departments and corporate wellness programs.

14-33 In the future, graduate students in exercise physiology will probably continue along the current narrow field of study.

14-34 Terms such as aerobic, training effect, and cholesterol are often misused and/or misunderstood by laypersons.

14-35 Although exercise factors in diabetes is an important area of study, it is not researched by exercise physiologists, but rather by biochemists and medical doctors.

14-36 Exercise physiologists in clinical practice do more applied research.

True-False Answers

1. T	7. F	13. F	19. T	25. F	31. T
2. F	8. T	14. F	20. F	26. F	32. F
3. T	9. F	15. T	21. F	27. T	33. F
4. F	10. F	16. F	22. T	28. T	34. F
5. T	11. T	17. T	23. T	29. T	35. F
6. T	12. F	18. F	24. F	30. F	36. T

Short Answer Questions

14-1 What is the study of the functioning of plants and animals and of the activities by which life is maintained and reproduced called?

ans: Physiology

14-2 What two areas of study have historically dominated exercise physiology research?

ans: a. How oxygen is utilized in the cardiovascular system
       b. The metabolic responses to exercise and training

14-3 What is spot reducing?

ans: When weight is lost in particular areas by use of heat or belts

14-4 What are four areas of study within basic exercise physiology?

ans: a. Environmental effects on exercise
       b. Disease and health
       c. Cardiovascular system
       d. Exercise biochemistry

14-5 What are three areas of study within clinical exercise physiology?

ans: a. Rehabilitation
       b. Prevention
       c. Age-related areas

14-6 What are the three major approaches to exercise physiology?

ans: a. Traditional cardiovascular and metabolic exercise physiology
       b. Exercise biochemistry
       c. Clinical exercise physiology, either cardiac rehabilitation or adult fitness

14-7 In what college departments could exercise physiologists be found?

ans: a. Sport sciences
       b. Physical education
       c. Physiology
       d. Cardiology
       e. Veterinary medicine
       f. Medicine

14-8 What is the name of a doctor trained to specialize in problems with the foot?

ans: A podiatrist

14-9 What will the future preparation for exercise physiologists probably be like?

ans: An effort will be made to train graduate students more completely in the sport sciences rather than narrowly in one field of study.

14-10 What are some erroneous beliefs that have been corrected by exercise physiology research?

ans: a. Athletes shouldn't drink water during practice on hot days.
        b. Girls/women shouldn't participate in vigorous sports.
        c. Swimmers shouldn't lift weights.
        d. Endurance work for children has negative effects.

14-11 What does work in cardiac rehabilitation involve?

ans: The assessment of cardiovascular functioning and prescriptive work in preventing cardiovascular trauma or rehabilitating persons who have experienced cardiovascular problems

14-12 What area of exercise physiology involves study at the cellular level?

ans: Exercise biochemistry

14-13 From an applied perspective, into what two areas of interest does exercise physiology typically divide?

ans: a. The enhancement of health and fitness with the concomitant prevention of debilitating disease (health-related fitness)
        b. The improvement of motor performance (motor performance fitness)

14-14 What was George Fitz's reaction to some of the outlandish claims made by the many developing systems prior to the beginning of the twentieth century?

ans: He spoke out against claims that could not be substantiated by research and called for the scientific study of exercise and physiology.

14-15 What effect has the large amount of research monies available for exercise physiology had?

ans: a. Much research has been produced.
       b. The stature of the field has been increased.
       c. The number of graduate students that can be supported has increased.

14-16 How does exercise physiology rank as far as popularity in the physical education subdisciplines?

ans: It is the most popular and best known.

14-17 What are some examples of aerobic activities that have a large accompanying literature available?

ans: a. Bicycling
       b. Cross-country skiing
       c. Jogging
       d. Walking

14-18 What are three of the major foci of small exercise physiology departments?

ans: a. Traditional cardiovascular and metabolic exercise physiology
       b. The newer exercise biochemistry
       c. Clinical exercise physiology in the form of cardiac rehabilitation or adult fitness

14-19 What are some of the related fitness professions for exercise physiology?

ans: a. Athletic training
       b. Cardiac rehabilitation
       c. Strength training
       d. Adult fitness professional

14-20 What would be the most direct prerequisite field to study in preparation for graduate work in exercise physiology?

ans: An undergraduate exercise science degree

14-21 What career would a masters degree program in exercise physiology typically prepare a person to do?

ans: a. Exercise specialist
        b. Exercise technician
        c. To work in a professional program such as cardiac rehabilitation or adult fitness

14-22 What are some of the problems associated with the field of exercise physiology?

ans: a. Research focus: clinical professionals would like more help and basic researchers feel that theory-oriented research pays better dividends
        b. The need for an interdisciplinary approach to investigate more fully the problems in exercise and sport
        c. Research is now only marginally associated with physical education

14-23 Why do basic exercise physiology researchers feel that theoretically based research pays higher dividends in the long run?

ans: Because it tends to focus on the underlying mechanisms rather that on applied problems.

14-24 Considering the newer socioecological view of health and fitness, what structures might have to be examined?

ans: Social, political, and economic structures that prevent portions of the population from gaining access to information, facilities, and programs related to fitness and health.

Chapter 15

Kinesiology and Biomechanics

If you have access to a high-speed film, it is interesting for students to watch a skill for several minutes that is performed in seconds at normal speed. Students are often unaware of how their equipment and events have changed as a result of this research field. The technical nature of the field should be explained carefully.

True-False Questions

15-1 Biomechanics is used almost exclusively in the college setting, as the performance of elite athletes is analyzed to give them a competitive edge.

15-2 Biomechanics is the study of how the muscular system moves the bony structure of the body.

15-3 The best procedure to improve sport skills is to have biomechanical advances precede the actual implementation of technique changes.

15-4 Biomechanics plays a role in equipment design, injury prevention and rehabilitation, and improved sport performance.

15-5 A biomechanist might work for a shoe company to design a shoe that eliminates foot problems for distance runners.

15-6 The motion that humans are capable of doing is determined exclusively by the type of the joint controlling that body part.

15-7 The shoulder joint is effective at extension/flexion movements.

15-8 Kinesiology is the course in which students learn to identify the actions of various joints and the muscles responsible for their movement.

15-9 A physical therapist might use knowledge of kinesiology to give a gradual exercise program designed to restore the full range of motion to a joint.

15-10 Movement possibilities always occur in pairs (i.e., flexion and extension of a joint).

15-11 A joint is capable of only one type of paired movement; i.e., wrist can only do flexion and extension.

15-12 Biomechanics is the study of human motion from the standpoint of physics.

15-13 Analysis of sports movements can be quite complex; for example, a golf swing has nearly one hundred forces acting on thirteen body segments.

15-14 When an implement is used to strike or receive an object, the implement and the object are not considered in the biomechanical analysis.

15-15 Motion, aerodynamics, and hydrodynamics are some of the physical principles applicable to biomechanical analysis.

15-16 The fields of kinesiology and biomechanics combine to form a coherent science of sport, although separately they are not utilized by researchers in the sport sciences.

15-17 Kinesiology has been a traditional field of study for physical education, but biomechanics as a specialized field of study did not really emerge until the mid-1960s.

15-18 Biomechanics developed out of the field of kinesiology and has recently begun to dominate the field.

15-19 The explosion of interest in sport and fitness has caused a decrease in the interest in biomechanics.

15-20 Laypersons and professionals are really not very knowledgeable about the mechanical or scientific aspects of technique.

15-21 The steady improvement of equipment is the direct result of a better understanding of biomechanics.

15-22 High-speed photography has been a major tool in the development of biomechanical research methods.

15-23 Electromyography is the technique of using a high-speed camera that slows down motion to the point at which it can be analyzed in great detail.

15-24 An athlete's slump can be detected by changes in an EMG pattern.

15-25 Computers can compare videotapes of athletes' performances to precise mathematical models of performance in an attempt to identify technical flaws.

15-26 High-speed photography, EMGs, and computer analysis of videotape are all examples of qualitative biomechanical analysis.

15-27 Mathematical models have led to the improvement of many sport skills, as is exemplified in the pole vault.

15-28 Physical education teachers use biomechanics when they observe a skill and give feedback to the students about correct execution and errors in the performance.

15-29 Pedagogical kinesiology emphasizes the critical elements and common errors of sport skill performance in practical situations rather than among elite athletes.

15-30 Biomechanists' knowledge is used exclusively in the fields of physical education and coaching at all levels.

15-31 A kinesiologist might study the difference in muscle potential in middle and long distance running.

15-32 Biomechanics is seen to have a bright future because of possible expansion into other fields such as child development and gerontology.

15-33 Most of the research done by biomechanists is of a highly practical nature with immediate application to physical education and coaching.

15-34 If a person chooses to specialize in kinesiology or biomechanics, a graduate degree, probably a doctorate, would be required.

15-35 The most typical background of someone going into the field of biomechanics is physics and math, due to the scientific nature of the discipline.

15-36 Most departments agree that undergraduate courses in biomechanics should emphasize the analysis of critical elements of a certain sport and subsequently give feedback to the performer.

15-37 Most money allocated to research in biomechanics comes from sources in sport and physical education.

15-38 A degree in kinesiology/biomechanics might typically include courses in engineering, research methods and statistics, and advanced mathematical courses.

15-39 A biomechanist working in the private sector is probably involved with the practical problems of equipment design and subsequent testing and evaluation of it.

15-40 There is continuing debate over the relative contributions made by quantitative and qualitative analysis.

True-False Answers

1. F	7. F	13. T	19. F	25. T	31. T	37. F
2. F	8. T	14. F	20. F	26. F	32. T	38. T
3. F	9. T	15. T	21. T	27. T	33. F	39. T
4. T	10. T	16. F	22. T	28. T	34. T	40. F
5. T	11. F	17. T	23. F	29. T	35. F	
6. F	12. T	18. T	24. T	30. F	36. F	

Short Answer Questions

15-1 What is kinesiology?

ans: The study of how the muscular system moves the bony structure of the body

15-2 Define biomechanics.

ans: The study of the human body as a mechanical system, utilizing principles and applications from physics

15-3 What are some of the goals that can accompany making the body move more efficiently? Give an example for each.

ans:　　a. Educational: a physical education teacher helping a student learn a motor skill
　　　　b. Competitive: a coach helping an elite athlete
　　　　c. Safety: a fitness instructor demonstrating correct lifting technique

15-4 Give examples of a biomechanical analysis both following and preceding newly introduced sport techniques.

ans:　　a. The Fosbury flop was performed in competition first and was analyzed afterward to show why it was effective.
　　　　b. Councilman analyzed the crawl to determine how to best perform the stroke. Swimmers began using that form successfully in competition.

15-5 What two anatomical features limit the range of human motion?

ans:　　a. The nature of the joint
　　　　b. The muscles moving the joint

15-6 What is the primary movement of the knee joint?

ans: Flexion and extension

15-7 Movement away from or toward the midline of the body is called:

ans: Abduction and adduction

15-8 What is another name for biomechanics?

ans: Mechanical kinesiology

15-9 What are the six physical principles applicable to biomechanical analysis?

ans:　　a. Motion
　　　　b. Force
　　　　c. Work and energy
　　　　d. Aerodynamics
　　　　e. Landing and striking
　　　　f. Hydrodynamics

15-10 What is a technique for recording the electrical impulses within muscles?

ans: Electromyography (EMG)

15-11 What are four modern technologies that have aided the scientific biomechanical analysis of sport?

ans:　　a. High-speed photography
　　　　b. Electromyography
　　　　c. Computer analysis
　　　　d. Mathematical modeling

15-12 The approach to biomechanics that emphasizes the recognition of the critical elements and common errors in sport skill performances is called

ans: Pedagogical kinesiology

15-13 What other fields are utilizing the knowledge of biomechanics?

ans:　　a. Physical therapy
　　　　b. Occupational therapy
　　　　c. Adapted physical education
　　　　d. Rehabilitative medicine

15-14 What sport would most benefit from the study of hydrodynamic effects?

ans: Swimming

15-15 What science is incorporated into the study of biomechanics?

ans: Physics

15-16 When did biomechanics as a specialized field of study begin to emerge?

ans: The mid-1960s

15-17 What field has contributed to a better understanding of equipment?

ans: Biomechanics

15-18 What is a quantitative biomechanical analysis?

ans: A method of analysis that utilizes sophisticated techniques to analyze sport movement. It is being used with increasing frequency to train elite athletes.

15-19 What is pedagogical kinesiology?

ans: An approach to biomechanics that emphasizes recognition of critical elements and common errors

15-20 Who would be most likely to utilize qualitative biomechanical analysis?

ans: The practitioner, i.e., the coach or teacher in the field

15-21 What other professions benefit from application of biomechanical knowledge?

ans: a. Physical therapy
       b. Occupational therapy
       c. Adapted physical education
       d. Rehabilitative medicine

15-22 What are four areas of study within kinesiology and biomechanics?

ans: a. Kinesiology
       b. Quantitative biomechanics
       c. Qualitative biomechanics
       d. Equipment

15-23 What are some career possibilities for a person trained in biomechanics?

ans: a. Research and teaching at a university or college
       b. Solve problems of product design, testing, and evaluation in the private sector
       c. Work with national sport teams

15-24 What level of degree is required to work as a kinesiologist or a biomechanist?

ans: Doctorate

15-25 Why is there concern that biomechanists receive research monies from sources whose concerns are not at all related to sport and physical education?

ans: There is some danger that kinesiologists and biomechanists will become more and more distanced from sport and physical education.

Chapter 16

Motor Learning, Control, and Development

Students who feel confident in their ability to coach a teenager are often brought up short when confronted with their inability to teach an unskilled child—a good confrontation to introduce them to the importance of these fields. A question like "what do you have to know to help a young child develop skill?" is a good entry.

True-False Questions

16-1 The field of motor control eventually expanded to include motor learning and motor development.

16-2 Motor learning, control, and development have all evolved historically from the field of psychology.

16-3 Motor development is a relatively permanent change in the performance of a motor skill that is the result of experience and/or practice.

16-4 Because most motor skill tasks initially involve the perception of an object, the acquisition of these skills is sometimes referred to as perceptual motor learning.

16-5 A major focus of motor control research is the influence by the nervous system in the muscular system to produce skilled movement.

16-6 The field of motor development looks at the aspects of motor skill from a learning rather than a hereditary standpoint.

16-7 Motor development researchers have identified environmental influences that affect the species, not just the individual.

16-8 While historically motor development had a major focus on developmental changes in infancy and childhood, it now encompasses the total lifespan of development, including aging.

16-9 Teachers and coaches are considered to be direct, applied motor learning practitioners.

16-10 Elementary and adapted physical education teachers both directly apply knowledge generated in the research field of motor development.

16-11 Cognitive and emotional development are closely related to motor development in young children as exploration of the world and sensory development all depend on movement.

16-12 Research done by motor development specialists suggests that systematic development of skill and fitness programs should not begin prior to age five.

16-13 Motor skill acquisition study began in the late nineteenth century when psychologists studied this topic on infrahuman subjects.

16-14 Much motor skill research occurred during and after World War II as a direct result of the poor physical condition of draftees.

16-15 When the discipline of physical education was created in the 1960s, motor learning emerged as one of the subdiscipline areas of study.

16-16 Early motor skill researchers tried to manipulate environmental variables to determine optimal practice schedules.

16-17 As researchers started studying the processes underlying motor development, fields such as neurophysiology, neuropsychology, and biomechanics were necessary for understanding.

16-18 Longitudinal studies, where different children of a given age are measured and tested for several years, are popular ways of studying growth and development.

16-19 Because of elementary physical education, researchers and practitioners have started studying developing motor behavior, such as jumping, throwing, and catching.

16-20 As children develop and learn, they must be treated as mini-adults so that adequate motor skill and fitness levels will develop as they mature.

16-21 Motor development at the graduate level is highly specialized, having links with experimental psychology and neuropsychology.

16-22 Motor development research has revealed much about the advantages of early physical education experiences, tracing adult fitness problems to habits established in early childhood.

16-23 Because of the popular interest in the topic of early childhood and infant motor and fitness training, the risk of myth and misinformation is greatly diminished.

16-24 Knowledge of motor development and learning is spreading to other fields as might be evidenced by architects and industrial technologists consulting a motor development specialist to design appropriate play spaces and equipment for children.

16-25 The field of motor development is expected to enlarge as issues of child care and early childhood education are addressed by state and/or federal legislation.

16-26 Motor learning and control specialists are usually found in governmental positions doing research and advisors to the department of education as well as other agencies.

16-27 Motor learning, development, and control differ from other "physical education professions" in that degrees in these areas are typically found at the undergraduate level.

16-28 Motor development training is typically tied to either a pedagogical or a sport science emphasis.

16-29 Most physical education majors have taken at least one class focusing on motor development/motor learning.

16-30 Much of the research done in motor learning is of direct benefit to a physical education teacher or coach.

16-31 As research and theory in motor learning have become more sophisticated, they increasingly address application problems in physical education and sport.

16-32 Basic research in motor development tends to address problems of a theoretical rather than an applied nature.

16-33 Motor development has addressed questions on influence of heredity or environment, producing rather convincing evidence that the latter has greater importance than the former.

16-34 Motor development will probably extend its research to problems associated with gerontology with decrements in motor performance as the main emphasis.

True-False Answers

1. F	6. F	11. T	16. T	21. F	26. F	31. F
2. T	7. F	12. F	17. T	22. T	27. F	32. T
3. F	8. T	13. T	18. F	23. F	28. T	33. F
4. T	9. F	14. F	19. T	24. T	29. T	34. T
5. T	10. T	15. T	20. F	25. T	30. F	

Short Answer Questions

16-1 What is motor control?

ans: The study of underlying processes controlling motor performance. The major focus of this area is how the nervous system controls the muscular system to produce skilled movement.

16-2 What is motor learning?

ans: A relatively permanent change in the performance of a motor skill resulting from experience and/or practice

16-3 What is the field that focuses both on total development of the individual and specifically on aspects of motor skill performance that are the result of heredity rather than learning?

ans: Motor development

16-4 What are the two ways heredity can be viewed?

ans: a. Specific to the individual
      b. Specific to the species

16-5 What fields have contributed to knowledge in the area of motor control?

ans: a. Neuropsychology
      b. Neurophysiology
      c. Cognitive psychology
      d. Biomechanics
      e. Computer science

16-6 Into what two fields can motor development be divided?

ans: a. Growth
      b. Perceptual-motor development

16-7 Why have professionals been concerned with the developmental stages persons go through as they move from infancy to adulthood?

ans: Because a major part of learning motor skills occurs from infancy through adolescence

16-8 Define the term "learning."

ans: A relatively permanent change in performance resulting from experience and/or practice

16-9 Why is the term perceptual motor learning used in place of motor learning?

ans: Motor skill tasks initially involve the perception of an object (usually visual perception) before the skill is performed.

16-10 What new part of the total lifespan of development is the field of motor development now starting to investigate?

ans: Aging

16-11 Who could be considered to be indirect applied motor learning practitioners?

ans: Teachers and coaches

16-12 What two types of teachers benefit directly from motor development research?

ans: a. Elementary physical education teachers
         b. Adaptive physical educators

16-13 How are cognitive and emotional development closely related to motor development at the early stages in a child's development?

ans: Exploration of the child's world, as well as sensory development, is dependent on movement. New knowledge is dependent upon the mastery of motor skills.

16-14 When did the most important growth for the field of motor learning occur and what was its purpose?

ans: The period of growth was during and just after World War II. Researchers were working on perceptual and motor skill acquisition projects associated with the war effort.

16-15 What are some of the research issues addressed during the time when motor learning emerged as one of the subdisciplines of physical education?

ans: a. Massed vs. distributed practice schedules
         b. The type and amount of feedback provided a learner
         c. Motivational variables

16-16 What journals are associated with the field of motor development that were begun in the 1960s?

ans: a. *Perceptual and Motor Skills*
       b. *Journal of Motor Behavior*

16-17 To what did the research focus of motor development shift during the 1970s, which led to the field of motor control?

ans: Researchers started examining the underlying processes that accompany the more visible task attributes of motor learning.

16-18 What two fields are considered equal partners in the general area of perceptual motor development?

ans: a. Motor learning
       b. Motor control

16-19 What *types* of studies are most famous in growth and development research?

ans: Longitudinal studies

16-20 What motor development behaviors have been studied by researchers and practitioners?

ans: a. Walking
       b. Climbing
       c. Jumping
       d. Throwing
       e. Catching

16-21 In what type of course would an undergraduate probably study motor control?

ans: Within a motor learning course

16-22 To which teaching fields does motor development have strong direct links?

ans: a. Early childhood education
       b. Elementary physical education
       c. Adapted physical education

16-23 What risks are associated when a field becomes a "popular" area of interest?

ans: Fads and misinformation

16-24 What are five examples of fields outside the realm of physical education that would have interest in motor learning, control, and development research?

ans: a. Architecture
        b. Physical rehabilitation
        c. Gerontology
        d. Early childhood education
        e. Industrial technology

16-25 Why is the field of motor development seen to be at the beginning stages of a period of substantial growth?

ans: During the next decade major legislation supporting child care and early childhood education will emerge at both the federal and state levels. Expertise and information available in motor development will be necessary when this happens.

16-26 Of the three areas of motor development, learning, or control, which area would be most likely to find employment in private industry?

ans: Motor development

16-27 Which area might be combined with elementary physical education expertise on the university level?

ans: Motor development

16-28 What two paths might lead to specialization in motor learning and motor control?

ans: An undergraduate degree in physical education or psychology

16-29 With what field does motor learning have a strong historical link?

ans: Psychology

16-30 What is one of the problems with research and theory in motor learning and control?

ans: As it has become more sophisticated, it has grown away from practical application to sport coaching and physical education.

16-31 What is the nature/nurture question?

ans: Which has greater influence over development, heredity or environment?

Chapter 17

Sport Sociology

A good project is to assign the questions in Table 17.1 to small groups and have them respond based on their "sense" of the issue, and then to compare that to what is known. Myths will surface quickly. How and why myths develop and how they can be harmful is a good discussion entry. This is, again, an opportunity to address equity issues.

True-False Questions

17-1 Sport sociology looks at the social patterns or social organization of those involved with sport, rather than a specific individual or group.

17-2 Sport has become a fundamental part of the culture of organized, industrialized societies.

17-3 Sport sociology as a subdiscipline focuses not only on sport, but on the areas of play and games as well.

17-4 Children's play tends to be largely unregulated, while adult play is typically rule-governed.

17-5 Despite its rather recent beginnings in the early 1960s, sport sociology is today firmly established as one of the important sport sciences.

17-6 Undergraduate physical education majors are often required to take sport sociology classes so as to better understand the role that sport plays in our culture and the issues pertaining to problems in sport.

17-7 Sport sociologists have addressed issues such as steroid use to build strength and underrepresentation of minorities in sport management.

17-8 Television commentators and sport writers tend to not pay much attention to sport sociology issues in favor of more dramatic and important ones.

17-9 Research has shown sport involvement to positively affect what is termed "character development."

17-10 Since sport sociologists are usually found in colleges and universities, the majority of their work is teaching, conducting research, and serving the community.

17-11 Sport sociologists often do clinical work directly with individual athletes or teams.

17-12 Graduate work in sport sociology requires an undergraduate degree in physical education to best understand the various sports in which future research will be done.

17-13 Sport sociology is researched from a value-free perspective, which is the traditional posture assumed by scientific inquiry.

17-14 Natural science inquiry methods are not often utilized in sport sociology so as to be more sensitive to some of the subjectivity that characterizes human behavior.

17-15 Sport sociologists study issues from a practical (applied) standpoint so as to best meet the needs of their clientele.

17-16 Critical theory represents a politically conservative approach to problems in sport and society.

True-False Answers

1. T	6. T	11. F	16. F
2. T	7. T	12. F	
3. T	8. F	13. F	
4. F	9. F	14. F	
5. T	10. T	15. F	

Short Answer Questions

17-1 What is sociology?

ans: The discipline in which the primary focus is the understanding of social organizations, the study of various social orders, and the analysis of regularities and irregularities in human social behavior

17-2 What are the characteristics of children's play?

ans: a. Free: no material interest or profit
       b. Separate: proceeds within its own proper boundaries of time and space
       c. Regulated: has its own rules
       d. Uncertain: the results and course of action are not predetermined
       e. Fictive
       f. Economically unproductive

17-3 What are two characteristics of adult play that differentiate it from that of children?

ans: a. Rule-governed
        b. Requires more preparation and training

17-4 What does sport sociology study?

ans: Social structure, social patterns, and social organization of groups engaged in sport

17-5 What are some of the issues in sport sociology?

ans: a. Overemphasis on winning in youth sport
        b. The forces that produce anorexia in young female athletes
        c. The use of steroids to build strength
        d. Use of drugs among professionals in sport
        e. Recruiting violations in collegiate sport
        f. Underrepresentation of minorities in sport management

17-6 What group of related terms best defines the interest areas of sport sociologists?

ans: a. Play
        b. Games
        c. Sport

17-7 What importance did Huizinga give to play?

ans: He felt that play was a fundamental impulse in human behavior.

17-8 What organization for sport sociologists is affiliated with AAHPERD?

ans: Sport Sociology Academy

17-9 During the 1970s, how were sport sociologists trained?

ans: Their programs were housed in departments of physical education with much coursework required in the cognate areas of sociology and social psychology.

17-10 How does the play of a child differ from that of an adult?

ans: Child's play is spontaneous, carefree, loose, and changeable, although it is governed by rules that children constantly change. Adult play is more typically rule governed and requires more preparation and training.

17-11 What sport sociology topics were of interest to the general public in the 1970s?

ans: a. The plight of the black athlete
        b. Recruiting violations in collegiate sport

17-12 Why do many undergraduate physical education programs require at least one course in sport sociology?

ans: Teachers, coaches, and other sport/fitness professionals need to understand the role that sport plays in culture, the ways in which persons are socialized in and through sport, and what issues pertain to problems in sport.

17-13 Why must topics such as character building in sport be studied?

ans: Not all sport experiences build character in a positive manner. One needs to find out what influences in sport participation have positive effects on character as well as those that have negative effects. When this is known, the positive influences can be emphasized in children's sport as the negative ones are minimized.

17-14 Where do sport sociologists primarily work, and what are their duties?

ans: Sport sociologists are almost always employed in academic positions in colleges and universities where they teach, do research, and provide service to the university and surrounding communities.

17-15 Do sport sociologists work directly with athletes or teams?

ans: Although the research done is often field based, there is no "clinical" sport sociology component as in sport psychology.

17-16 By what two paths do people typically become sport sociologists?

ans: a. Undergraduate major in physical education and graduate study at a school that
            has a sport sociology specialization
        b. Undergraduate major in sociology and graduate training in that area with a
            department that had a strong sport sociology component

17-17 What is meant by "value-free" research?

ans: That which is objective and free from a pre-research bias

17-18 What controversy surrounds the research methods used by sport sociologists?

ans: Some feel that the objective methods utilized from the natural sciences will produce the best results, whereas others prefer the greater amounts of data produced by subjective methodology.

17-19 What are the three issues of greatest debate in sport sociology?

ans: a. Value vs. value-free research
         b. Subjective vs. objective research
         c. Theory-oriented vs. action-oriented research

Chapter 18

Sport Psychology

Starting with common media concepts like momentum, "choking," and team cohesiveness is useful. Students will have strong opinions. Descriptions of some of the clinical treatments—mental imagery, coping, etc.—help to establish the technical nature of this specialization. The question "who is better, the trained psychologist with an interest in sport, or the trained sportsperson with knowledge of psychology?" often provokes debate.

True-False Questions

18-1 A clinical sport psychologist would study the biophysical, psychosocial, and intrapersonal variables that influence the performance of athletes and teams.

18-2 Academic sport psychologists tend to be university professors working in departments of psychology, physical education, or sport psychology.

18-3 A clinical sport psychologist might travel with a national team to provide treatments to improve the performance of athletes.

18-4 A sport psychologist must pass a national exam in order to obtain a license before he or she can practice.

18-5 Practicing sport psychologists may have preparation in that area, be clinical psychologists, or have been trained in counseling psychology.

18-6 Sport psychologists differ from regular psychologists in that they study and/or give treatment to the behaviors of individuals or groups rather than working only with the mental aspects of performance and competition.

18-7 The early history of sport psychology was tied closely with that of motor learning, as people with a background in psychology could relate to both fields.

18-8 When the North American Society for the Psychology of Sport and Physical Activity (NASPSPA) formed in 1968, the subdisciplines of motor learning and sport psychology divided to form their own study areas.

18-9 The discipline movement in physical education contributed strongly to the development of a sport psychology area.

18-10 Because of the popularity of the subject areas, several schools have developed undergraduate degrees in sport psychology.

18-11 A good way to differentiate between the two types of sport psychologists would be to say that academic sport psychologists contribute to the knowledge base of the field, whereas practicing sport psychologists do not.

18-12 Early sport psychology research looked at the personalities of various types of athletes.

18-13 The current focus of research in sport psychology is to use theories from the parent field of psychology and see how they apply to the sport setting.

18-14 A question typical of the psychobiological topic area might be, "Can sport exercise help to replace chemical dependency?"

18-15 An academic sport psychologist typically works in the academic setting, teaching classes and conducting research, but has no contact with athletic teams except for research studies.

18-16 A practicing sport psychologist might have a performance enhancement role doing such things as teaching the athlete to relax during competition or mentally rehearsing positive performances.

18-17 Desensitization is when an athlete is taught to mentally rehearse successful performance just prior to beginning the performance.

18-18 Coping strategies try to anticipate events that might intrude in pre-performance time or during performance, and then involve developing and rehearsing behavioral strategies to cope with and overcome these incidents.

18-19 Cue-controlled relaxation and relations training are different terms for the same phenomenon.

18-20 Sport psychologists who counsel their athletes usually work with personal problems, thus allowing the athlete to devote full attention to the athletic performance.

18-21 Practicing sport psychologists can observe potential problems such as those among players or between the player and coach and counsel the people involved before real problems arise.

18-22 In order to be a sport psychologist, the person must have been trained as either a clinical psychologist or a counseling psychologist.

18-23 The Psychological Advisory Committee of the United States Olympic Committee has recently defined minimum educational and experiential requirements for sport psychologists trying to obtain a license to practice.

18-24 The vast majority of academic and practicing sport psychologists have doctoral degrees.

18-25 The American Association of State Psychology board has recommended that all doctoral programs include minimally three years of full-time graduate study with at least one year of continuous full-time residency at the university.

18-26 The requirements for clinical or counseling psychologists are determined by the individual states granting the license.

18-27 Sport psychologists agree that academic sport psychologists should utilize theory and research from the parent discipline of psychology instead of taking the time to develop the theory from research done in the field of sport.

18-28 European sport psychology is practiced by the coaches rather than a separate individual.

18-29 Sport psychologists of the future will probably have additional training in other sport sciences, such as biomechanics, sport nutrition, or motor development.

18-30 Whereas the early history of sport psychology has dealt with youth sport, the future will probably include more attention to the needs of the elite athletes and coaches.

True-False Answers

1. F	6. F	11. F	16. T	21. T	26. T
2. T	7. T	12. T	17. F	22. F	27. F
3. T	8. F	13. F	18. T	23. F	28. T
4. F	9. T	14. T	19. F	24. T	29. T
5. T	10. F	15. F	20. T	25. T	30. F

Short Answer Questions

18-1 What is the study of human behavior called?

ans: Psychology

18-2 The field that applies psychology to issues and problems in sport is called:

ans: Sport psychology

18-3 What are the two major sub-groups within sport psychology?

ans: a. The academic study of sport psychology
b. Clinical practice of sport psychology

18-4 What are the two approaches to treatment in sport psychology? What does each group study?

ans: a. Treatment of the mental aspects of sport performance and competition. They look at why people behave as they do.
b. Work with the behavior(s) of individuals and groups. They try to help people behave more effectively.

18-5 What have been the three phases of sport psychology research?

ans: a. Phase one looked at personalities of various groups of athletes.
b. Phase two borrowed theories from the parent field of psychology and tested them in the sport settings. It also looked at interactional approaches and formulations of operant conditioning models for sport.
c. Phase three focused on developing information and theory directly derived from sport. It also looked at the development and refinement of a number of psychological skills and strategies used to enhance sport performance.

18-6 What are the four topic areas of academic sport psychology?

ans: a. Psychophysiological approaches
b. Psychobiological approaches
c. Self-regulation
d. Social psychology

18-7 What are the two roles, direct and indirect, that a practicing sport psychologist can fill?

ans: a. Directly improve performance: performance enhancement role
b. Indirectly: by counseling athletes to help them overcome problems

18-8 What is one source of controversy in American sport psychology?

ans: The field has become too academic or too theory oriented.

18-9 When athletes are taught to feel tension in muscles and learn how to control release of tension, this is called:

ans: Relaxation training

18-10 What is cue-controlled relaxation?

ans: A relaxation strategy that is tied to a word cue that allows the athlete to say the word to himself or herself and induce relaxation

18-11 Describe the process of desensitization.

ans: Gradually reducing anxiety caused in specific competitive situations by teaching the athlete to relax while imaging a series of increasingly adversive competitive situations

18-12 What is mental imaging?

ans: Teaching athletes to mentally rehearse successful performance just prior to beginning the performance

18-13 Give some examples of coping strategies.

ans: Rehearsing the specific procedures to follow when going to compete in a foreign land and how to cope with language, security, time, and food incidents.
        Practicing what to do during an event if certain situations arise.

18-14 When an athlete imagines a model doing a particular performance as a means to help the athlete acquire that skill or ability, this is called:

ans: Covert modeling

18-15 What is a broad goal of academic sport psychologists?

ans: To identify factors that are particularly important in sport settings, especially those related to sport performance

18-16 In what departments might you find academic sport psychologists?

ans: a. Psychology
        b. Physical education
        c. Sport psychology

18-17 What is the purpose of the clinical sport psychologist?

ans: To utilize psychological interventions to improve the performance of an athlete or to increase the psychological well-being of the athlete

18-18 What effect does absence of licensing have on sport psychologists?

ans: They come from varied backgrounds. The training and preparation is quite different depending on their background.

18-19 Where did the predominant development of sport psychology occur in the 1970s?

ans: In the colleges and universities within physical education departments

18-20 What will likely determine how sport psychologists will be trained in the future?

ans: Whether or not they are certified or licensed

18-21 What are the five types of sport psychology literature?

ans: a. Research journals
        b. Conference proceedings
        c. Textbooks and books on readings
        d. Coaching texts
        e. Popular books

18-22 What is the work of academic sport psychologists?

ans: They study the psychological aspects of sport performance.

18-23 In what capacity do practicing sport psychologists function?

ans: They work directly with athletes.

18-24 What are two ways in which a counseling psychologist might help athletes?

ans: a. Cope with the stress in their personal lives
        b. Work with the relationships among athletes on a team and between athletes and their coaches

18-25 What are the three primary paths that can lead to a career in sport psychology?

ans: a. Graduate training in sport psychology
        b. Training as a clinical psychologist
        c. Training as a counseling psychologist

18-26 Why is licensing and certification an issue in sport psychology?

ans: Because specialized skills are being offered to clients for a fee.

18-27 What is one of the reasons for the split in American sport psychology?

ans: People felt sport psychology had become too academic, too theory oriented, and not sufficiently grounded in the practice of sport.

18-28 By tradition, who learns sport psychology skills in Europe? Why?

ans: The coaches, so they can apply them directly to the team and athletes

18-29 If sport psychologists become more firmly anchored with sport sciences in the future, what type of ancillary training will be required?

ans: a. Sport biomechanics
         b. Sport nutrition
         c. Motor development

18-30 What area of sport has been understudied and relatively neglected in sport psychology?

ans: The areas of children's and youth sports, and individual athletes' total well being.

18-31 Sport psychology will likely be anchored in what area in the future?

ans: Sport sciences

Chapter 19

Sport Pedagogy

The research questions in 19.1 provide a good entry when students are asked to respond to them based on (a) their own experience and (b) their sense of the ideal teacher/coach. Differences between teaching and coaching provide interesting topics for discussion. It is also useful to explore whether students see major differences in preparing to be a teacher/coach educator as opposed to being a sport psychologist or sport biomechanist, especially in terms of the technical, scientific expertise needed.

True-False Questions

19-1 Children can be born with certain sport skills, and these children are referred to as "naturals."

19-2 Virtually all cultures, once they get beyond the subsistence stage of development, consider sport and physical education to be of enough importance to arrange programs through which these skills can be learned.

19-3 In the rest of the world except the United States, sport pedagogy encompasses coaching in community or club programs as well as physical education programs.

19-4 The term "pedagogy" in the phrase "sport pedagogy" refers to the actual act of teaching.

19-5 In the term "sport pedagogy," sport should be loosely defined to include competitive sport, leisure, and fitness activities as well.

19-6 The term "teacher education" is synonymous with "sport pedagogy" throughout the world.

19-7 A youth sport coach has many of the same problems and thus needs many of the same skills as a physical education teacher working in a school setting.

19-8 A sport pedagogy practitioner would be the person designated to implement the research from that as well as other sport fields.

19-9 The instruction phase of sport pedagogy deals with teacher interaction skills, assessment of performance and learning, and management/discipline issues related to teaching and coaching.

19-10 The field of curriculum tends to be almost exclusively of a theoretical nature, focusing on models.

19-11 Sport pedagogy is the only area where one will not see new faculty positions advertised in that specific discipline.

19-12 The fields of instruction and curriculum are usually separate with practitioners involved in instruction and researchers involved in curriculum.

19-13 Because the focus of physical education has been historically to train teachers, sport pedagogy is considered to be the oldest of the sport sciences.

19-14 The emergence of a discipline approach to physical education was in many ways a reaction to the low status of teacher education programs for that subject area.

19-15 Prior to the 1970s, virtually every college physical education teacher considered him/herself to be a teacher educator.

19-16 Physical education departments experimented with the possibility of alternate careers to accommodate the oversupply of physical education teachers, which in some respects helped lead to the development of the discipline approach.

19-17 Because of the subject area, sport pedagogy has developed a knowledge base quite different from that of regular teacher education research.

19-18 Sport pedagogy now has a national association, whose publication is called the *Journal of Teaching in Physical Education.*

19-19 AAHPERD has several affiliations that play an important role in the needs of specialized areas of physical education, most notably the National Association for Sport and Physical Education (NASPE) and the Council of Physical Education for Children (COPEC).

19-20 International sport pedagogists belong to the United States Association for Sport Pedagogy, as there are no organizations outside of the United States that publish research and host conferences.

19-21 Despite the push toward improving sport pedagogy, the content of current teacher education textbooks is much like that published a generation ago.

19-22 The demand for teacher education faculty is currently increasing due to retirement of current faculty and increasing demands for new physical educators.

19-23 Teacher behavior research might try to see behavior differences between elementary and secondary teachers.

19-24 Teacher effectiveness research might look at the problems encountered by first-year teachers.

19-25 Although teacher education research has begun to change the content of teacher and coach preparation programs, work with inservice teachers has not yet been affected.

19-26 Because of classroom management research, teachers and coaches know that using established managerial routines, which help keep management time low, is an effective teaching strategy.

19-27 Instructional teaching strategies have not benefited very much to date in physical education teacher effectiveness research.

19-28 Research in curriculum has progressed rapidly, as shown by the new curricular models of sport and fitness education.

19-29 A physical education teacher educator may teach sport skill classes to physical education majors, supervise student teachers, and teach methods of teaching classes on any given day.

19-30 Sport pedagogy is currently a doctoral specialization at many universities that usually requires an undergraduate degree in physical education and a minimum of three years of teaching experience.

19-31 A degree in sport pedagogy would probably include classes in teaching research, teacher education, supervision, and research methodology.

19-32 The fields of adaptive physical education and sport psychology are closely related to sport pedagogy, and students in all three areas would likely gain experience in the other fields as well.

19-33 One of the important issues in sport pedagogy is whether teachers will continue to be certified at the undergraduate level.

19-34 The push for teacher certification at the graduate level is mainly an effort to increase the starting salaries of new teachers, as those with masters degrees receive more money than those with only an undergraduate degree.

19-35 Teacher training at the graduate level for a physical education major would be easier than for other majors because of the extensive sport experiences of potential physical education majors.

True-False Answers

1. F	6. F	11. F	16. T	21. F	26. T	31. T
2. T	7. T	12. F	17. F	22. T	27. F	32. F
3. T	8. T	13. F	18. F	23. T	28. T	33. T
4. F	9. T	14. T	19. T	24. T	29. T	34. F
5. T	10. F	15. T	20. F	25. F	30. T	35. F

Short Answer Questions

19-1 What are the functions for the two types of sport pedagogists?

ans: a. Creation of new knowledge (research)
        b. Implementation of that knowledge (practice)

19-2 What are the two main areas into which sport pedagogy is typically divided?

ans: a. Instruction
        b. Curriculum

19-3 What are two reasons why the demand for teacher education faculty is increasing?

ans: a. Retirement of current PETE faculty
        b. Increased need for school physical education teachers

19-4 What five areas are currently being investigated within sport pedagogy?

ans: a. Teacher behavior
        b. Student behavior
        c. Teacher effectiveness
        d. Teacher issues
        e. Curriculum

19-5 What are the functions of sport pedagogists?

ans: a. Teach sport skills to physical education majors
        b. Teach methods classes
        c. Organize and supervise on-campus clinical experiences for preservice teachers
        d. Organize and supervise field-based experiences for preservice teachers
        e. Supervise student teachers
        f. Teach courses related to teacher preparation

19-6 By what two terms might sport pedagogy be referred to in the United States?

ans: a. Teacher education
      b. Curriculum and instruction

19-7 How do we know that sport is valued by cultures?

ans: Virtually all cultures, once they get beyond the subsistence stage of development, consider sport and physical education to be sufficiently important that they arrange programs for the young persons in the culture to acquire the skills and strategies of sport in their childhood and youth and improve them through practice and competition.

19-8 What is sport pedagogy?

ans: The study of the processes of teaching and coaching, the outcomes of such endeavors, and the content of fitness, physical education, and sport education programs

19-9 What has been the effect of not using the broader term "sport pedagogy" in the United States?

ans: The scope of school programs of physical education, teaching within school programs, and the content of the programs themselves have been restricted.

19-10 In most of the rest of the world, what does sport pedagogy encompass?

ans: Coaching in the community or in clubs and teaching physical education in the schools

19-11 What does pedagogy include beyond the act of teaching?

ans: a. Developing a program
      b. Planning for the implementation of that program
      c. Assessing the outcomes of the program

19-12 What is the risk of defining a sport pedagogy program too narrowly?

ans: It will be restricted solely to what goes on in school programs of physical education and neglect teaching/coaching in the community and club programs as well as lifelong involvement in sport, fitness, and physical education.

19-13 What issues might be examined in the field of instruction?

ans: a. Planning
        b. Teacher interaction skills
        c. The activities of students/players that contribute to learning
        d. The assessment of performance and learning
        e. The comparison of different teaching/coaching methods
        f. Management/discipline issues related to teaching and coaching

19-14 On what issues does the field of curriculum focus?

ans: a. The content of programs
        b. The goals that programs are or should be devoted to
        c. The manner in which programs are implemented
        d. The outcomes achieved within programs, especially as they relate to program
            goals

19-15 What factor contributed significantly to the development of the subdiscipline of sport pedagogy?

ans: Many subdisciplines were created in physical education largely as a reaction to the low status of physical education in university education departments. Sport pedagogy was a reaction to the development of other subdisciplines.

19-16 What publication represented an important milestone in the development of sport pedagogy?

ans: *Journal of Teaching in Physical Education*

19-17 In which national organization do most sport pedagogists have membership?

ans: American Alliance for Health, Physical Education, Recreation, and Dance (AAHPERD)

19-18 Give examples of topics that are treated differently in textbooks because of the knowledge gained from research in the past generation.

ans: a. Classroom management
        b. Discipline
        c. Instruction

19-19 As a result of sport pedagogy research, what motto could be used to replace the phrase "practice makes perfect"?

ans: Good practice makes perfect.

19-20 What types of jobs would a person trained at the doctoral level in sport pedagogy be capable of doing?

ans: a. Professor in a college or university
      b. Employment in a K–12 school as a department director
      c. A curriculum director for a school district
      d. A supervisor of physical education for a school district

19-21 What fields are closely related to sport pedagogy?

ans: a. Motor development
      b. Adaptive physical education

19-22 What is seen to be a major issue associated with sport pedagogy in America?

ans: Should teacher training occur at the graduate or undergraduate level?

19-23 What is the primary mission of sport pedagogy?

ans: Teacher education

19-24 According to Siedentop and Locke (1997), what is the criterion for judging the success of teacher education programs?

ans: That they contribute directly to the development, maintenance, and dissemination of high quality school physical education programs.

Chapter 20

The Sport Humanities

Watching a film, reading excerpts from books, reviewing sculpture and painting, or reading poetry all make for good entries to this area of specialization. Asking students to respond to what they see as most beautiful in sport or of most value in sport sometimes serves well as a discussion focus for the humanistic specializations.

True-False Questions

20-1 The sport humanities are comprised of sport history and sport literature.

20-2 Until recent times, sports literature was not a major focus of the sport humanities.

20-3 By definition, history as a field of study is a description of past events.

20-4 According to Adelman, interpretive-comparative historical investigations represent a more mature development of the field than narrative-descriptive ones.

20-5 Most sport history works are of the interpretive-comparative nature.

20-6 Narrative-descriptive historical books provide a description of events that occurred during a given period and relates these to happenings in other times.

20-7 Metaphysics is the branch of philosophy that studies questions about values.

20-8 How knowledge is acquired is the field of epistemology, whereas the relationship of ideas composes the study of logic.

20-9 One of the reasons philosophy is difficult to understand is that there is no set methodology with which to investigate philosophical problems.

20-10 Philosophy as a first-order activity is a discipline with a unique set of problems that are classified within four branches: metaphysics, axiology, epistemology, and logic.

20-11 By definition, philosophic points of view are held only by those sport professionals who are trained in philosophic logic.

20-12 Analytic philosophy refers to general principles that provide guidelines for behavior in practical activities.

20-13 Speculative philosophy focuses on arguments that extend beyond the limits of scientific or factual origin.

20-14 An example of a question asked in analytic philosophy might be: "What various meanings does the term 'fitness' have in current and popular scientific literature?"

20-15 J. B. Nash, Rosalind Cassidy, and Delbert Oberteuffer were best known for their philosophical writings as they contributed to the physical education profession.

20-16 Sports literature encompasses fiction, poetry, and films that have a permanent value due to their excellence of form, their emotional effect, and their ability to provide insights about the human condition.

20-17 By definition, books about championship teams, written either by ghost writers or in collaboration with a popular athlete, have literary merit because of their wide sales and consequent influence on the general public.

20-18 The development of sport history, sport philosophy, and sport literature is of a recent nature, part of the general trend toward a discipline of physical education.

20-19 Of Eyler's (1965) three periods, sport history now appears to be in the approbatory period.

20-20 Eyler's approbatory period is characterized by a rich and full body of knowledge covering the major periods of history, the full range of sports, and utilizing the interpretive-comparative approach.

20-21 Sport philosophers who work within the Philosophic Society for the Study of Sport (PSSS) have been careful to include both first-order and second-order activities so as to meet the needs of all those who are interested in this subject area.

20-22 The major focus of the *Journal of Sport Literature* is sport and fitness.

20-23 The study of sport humanities would be equated with a liberal arts approach to educating students.

20-24 The growth and success of the sport humanities is attributed to the high rate of employability of students who select this education emphasis.

20-25 Investigations in the sport humanities can help to focus and clarify issues such as how we as sport, fitness, and physical educational professionals fit into the big picture.

20-26 The study of sport humanities is not important as a general area of study but rather should be viewed as an area of specialization for graduate students.

20-27 Those studying sport humanities come almost entirely from those who have studied sport and physical education as undergraduates.

20-28 Because sport humanities departments tend to be small, people in that subject area are called upon to teach specialized courses in that field.

20-29 A person desiring work in the sport humanities could have an undergraduate major in physical education and then at the graduate level major in history, philosophy, or literature with a sport emphasis.

20-30 A doctoral degree is probably a prerequisite to work in a college or university in the field of sport humanities.

20-31 The major problem in sport humanities is the lack of qualified applicants to fill various university and college positions.

20-32 A second major problem in the sport humanities is ignorance of the subject area on the part of sports writers and sport commentators.

20-33 Sport philosophers have tended to focus on academic philosophy rather than to speak to issues of general concern to practitioners in the profession.

20-34 The fact that the work of professional philosophy specialists is too irrelevant to professional life suggests that interest in philosophic issues is waning.

20-35 The sport humanities have been expanding their focus and now address issues in sport, fitness, and physical education.

True-False Answers

1. F	6. F	11. F	16. T	21. F	26. F	31. F
2. T	7. F	12. F	17. F	22. F	27. F	32. T
3. F	8. T	13. T	18. T	23. T	28. F	33. T
4. T	9. F	14. T	19. F	24. F	29. T	34. F
5. F	10. T	15. T	20. T	25. T	30. T	35. F

Short Answer Questions

20-1 What fields comprise the sport humanities?

ans: a. Sport history
        b. Sport philosophy
        c. Sport literature

20-2 Give five examples of how sport is influencing our culture.

ans: a. 15–20% of newspaper space is devoted to sport
         b. Endless hours of television coverage
         c. Sport is a part of the evening news
         d. International events are covered by television for extended periods of time
             (Olympics, Wimbledon)
         e. A national "championship" seems to bring the nation to a halt
         f. Sport and fitness sections in the bookstores are among the largest
         g. Many specialized magazines
         h. Weekly sport coverage by a national magazine *(Sports Illustrated)*

20-3 What is a narrative-descriptive book?

ans: A historical book that describes what went on during a given period

20-4 What is an interpretive-comparative book?

ans: A book that describes and interprets historical events and compares them to other periods of time

20-5 A branch of philosophy that addresses questions about the nature of reality is called

ans: Metaphysics

20-6 What is axiology?

ans: A branch of philosophy that studies values

20-7 What does the study of logic encompass?

ans: The relationship of ideas

20-8 What is the branch of philosophy that looks at how knowledge is gained?

ans: Epistemology

20-9 What is the term for a philosophy that focuses on arguments that extend beyond the limits of scientific or factual knowledge?

ans: Speculative philosophy

20-10 What are the three categories into which philosophical concerns fall?

ans: a. Speculative philosophy
        b. Normative philosophy
        c. Analytic philosophy

20-11 What is normative philosophy?

ans: A philosophy that refers to general principles that provide guidelines for behavior in practical activities

20-12 Which philosophy deals with the clarification of words or concepts?

ans: Analytic philosophy

20-13 What are the three periods through which the field of sport history would develop as predicted by Eyler in 1965?

ans: a. Awakening period
        b. Fledgling period
        c. Approbatory period

20-14 In which of these periods is the field of sport history currently placed?

ans: Fledgling period

20-15 Explain what first-order and second-order philosophic activities are.

Ans: Philosophy as a first-order activity is a discipline with a unique set of problems classified in the four branches of metaphysics, axiology, epistemology, and logic.
        Philosophy as a second-order activity refers to thinking creatively and logically about problems that belong to areas outside philosophy itself.

20-16 What broader view of history must be taken rather than just considering it a description of past events?

ans: History is a bridge connecting the past with the present and pointing the road to the future.

20-17 According to Adelman, which category of historical investigations represents a more mature development of the field?

ans: Interpretive-comparative

20-18 What did the organization of the Philosophic Society for the Study of Sport (PSSS) represent?

ans: The marriage of sport and philosophy

20-19 What three physical education fields have their roots in the humanities rather than in the sciences?

ans: a. Sport history
        b. Sport philosophy
        c. Sport literature

20-20 What are some of the major problems within the field of sport humanities?

ans: a. Departments are too small and in constant danger of losing what little they have
        b. Uninformed sports writers and sport commentators
        c. Sport philosophers have tended to focus on academic philosophy rather than the issues of concern to practitioners
        d. Focus on sport with little attention given to fitness and physical education

20-21 When is a piece considered to have literary value?

ans: Books, poetry, and films that have a permanent value due to their excellence of form, their emotional effect, and their ability to provide insights about the human condition

20-22 What journal is published by the PSSS?

ans: *Journal of the Philosophic Society for the Study of Sport*

20-23 How do the philosophical interests of members of PSSS differ from those of AAHPERD members who indicate an interest in philosophy?

ans: PSSS members approach philosophy as a first-order activity, whereas AAHPERD members are interested in philosophy as a second-order activity.

20-24 What journal is published by those interested in sport literature?

ans: *Arete: The Journal of Sport Literature*

20-25 Why haven't the sport humanities grown?

ans: There are few programs that emphasize them, and the trend has been toward vocationally oriented programs rather than those emphasizing a liberal arts approach.

20-26 How does the general public interpret many of the things done by physical education professionals?

ans: Through the sport humanities

20-27 Why is the study of sport humanities important for physical education professionals?

ans: It stimulates interest in sport as well as promotes one's ability to think critically about the work one does as well as extend one's appreciation for the importance and complexity of that work.

20-28 What do people in the sport humanities do?

ans: They are mostly employed in academic positions in colleges and universities.

20-29 What credentials are required for an academic specialist in the field of sport humanities?

ans: A doctorate with a strong concentration in the parent area (history, philosophy, or literature)

20-30 What problem transcends all three areas of sport humanities?

ans: The lack of focus on fitness and physical education

20-31 What is the main problem within the sport humanities?

ans: They are too small and are not sufficiently represented in undergraduate and graduate curricula in teacher education and the sport sciences.

Chapter 21

Relationships to Allied Fields

Discussing allied fields from a futuristic perspective is interesting and useful. How should they relate in the future? How will specialization help or harm these relationships and the services provided by each field? What are the job opportunities locally? Who occupies those jobs, and what training do they have?

True-False Questions

21-1 The fragmentation of the profession of health, physical education, and recreation has been the direct result of specialization within the respective fields.

21-2 The distinctions between health, education, and recreation professionals are seldom noticed by most of the people for whom they provide services.

21-3 Most professionals within the fields of health, education, and recreation are seldom noticed by most of the people for whom they provide services.

21-4 Recreation programs are considered to be a necessary part of an overall quality lifestyle, and an active, healthy leisure life is thought to have restorative power.

21-5 As a profession develops, the tendency is toward more professional preparation and implementation of certification standards.

21-6 Although a number of specializations have developed in recreation, members have remained affiliated with AAHPERD, the largest professional organization in the field of recreation.

21-7 The American Association for Leisure and Recreation is the member organization for recreation in AAHPERD.

21-8 The largest areas of growth in the recreation and leisure services industry in the recent past have been in government agencies and commercial recreation enterprises.

21-9 One of the factors in the growth of recreation and leisure services has been the willingness of people to spend discretionary income on these pastimes.

21-10 Accreditation requires that people earn a license to practice their profession following a procedure outlined by state legislation.

21-11 Program accreditation now exists widely in the recreation and leisure services professions, which helps ensure that personnel directing programs have competencies that promote safety and appropriate programming.

21-12 Stress management is a specialized field that tends to bring the recreation and health professions together.

21-13 As adults tend to stay active in more vigorous activities, preparation for leisure is no longer recognized as a goal in school programs.

21-14 If lifespan sport, fitness, and physical education are to become more of a reality for a larger percentage of the population, interrelationships among the fields will need to develop and strengthen.

21-15 Americans from all income brackets have taken health more seriously in the past several decades than ever before.

21-16 The focus of the health professions has remained a remedial or medical approach, as is evidenced by the high costs of hospital stays and visits to doctors.

21-17 Americans are living longer and the "senior" cohort age group is becoming a strong political and social force in American society.

21-18 Traditionally the primary focus of the health professions has been the education of children, and youth and health education has been and still remains the strongest force in the emerging health professions.

21-19 The school health education program has grown steadily more important and increasingly separate from physical education.

21-20 Many states have enacted laws requiring that health education be taught in schools. Some laws even specify the grade levels at which health education is taught.

21-21 The American Heart Association and the Lung Association are two examples of government programs that generate financial support for research and program development.

21-22 The strongest recent growth in the health enhancement industry has occurred in the school health education and community health programs.

21-23 Predictions are that the work place will become a major provider of health, recreation, and fitness.

21-24 Estimates are that by 1990, more than one-fourth of all American corporations will provide employee recreation and fitness programs.

21-25 The major impetus for worksite health enhancement programs has been the tax breaks offered by the federal government.

21-26 Poor health among employees leads to higher absenteeism and lessened worker productivity.

21-27 The private sector of the health enhancement industry is highly regulated, requiring health professionals to have certifications and licenses.

21-28 School health educators are certified and licensed to teach in the same way all teachers are.

21-29 There is no certification in community health programs, although many colleges and universities have undergraduate degree specializations in community health.

21-30 The positive aspect of the wellness revolution has increased the fitness levels in children as well as made parents more knowledgeable about health needs for children so that they may encourage proper eating habits.

21-31 Today, fewer people smoke and a smaller percentage start smoking.

21-32 By making a few relatively simple decisions, an individual can greatly reduce risk for degenerative disease.

21-33 Dance has only recently become a significant human activity in world cultures.

21-34 Dance has been utilized as a means of expression, as is evidenced by the growing use of dance therapy.

21-35 Dance in physical education has been, and continues to be, severely restricted and limited in scope.

21-36 Most physical education teachers have traditionally had little or no dance training and as a result have been reluctant to teach it.

21-37 A movement known as the "discipline-based arts education" focuses on the technique of art but also has an emphasis on understanding the arts.

21-38 Dance curriculums now emphasize being both the performer and consumer (or audience) of dance.

21-39 Folk and ballet remain the two strongest dance forms in college and university dance departments.

21-40 Curriculums are being developed at several major universities that will enable beginning professionals to function well in any of the health, recreation, or dance fields.

True-False Answers

1. T	7. T	13. F	19. T	25. F	31. T	37. T
2. T	8. F	14. T	20. T	26. T	32. T	38. T
3. F	9. T	15. F	21. F	27. F	33. F	39. F
4. T	10. F	16. F	22. F	28. T	34. T	40. F
5. T	11. T	17. T	23. T	29. T	35. F	
6. F	12. T	18. F	24. T	30. F	36. T	

Short Answer Questions

21-1 What is recreation?

ans: Activities or experiences chosen voluntarily and done during leisure time for the satisfaction they provide the individuals and groups involved

21-2 What are the four components through which the recreation and leisure services industry delivers its programs to groups and individuals?

ans: a. Government agencies
        b. Voluntary organizations
        c. Private membership groups
        d. Commercial recreation enterprises

21-3 What are the five major components through which the services of the health enhancement industry are delivered?

ans: a. School health education
        b. Government and community health programs
        c. Non-profit health organizations
        d. Worksite health programs
        e. Private sector entrepreneurial programs

21-4 In what four ways does poor health among employees cut profit margins for industry?

ans: a. Absenteeism
        b. Lessened productivity
        c. Reduced morale among employees
        d. Increased costs of worker compensation programs

21-5 What are the ways in which an individual can greatly reduce (or increase) his or her risk for degenerative disease?

ans: a. Smoking
      b. Alcohol use
      c. Diet
      d. Exercise
      e. Seat belt use
      f. Periodic screening for major diseases

21-6 What are some of the contributions dance can make to our culture?

ans: a. Educational
      b. A means of expression
      c. Important to fitness
      d. An expression of the popular culture

21-7 Who would be unlikely to notice many distinctions between the fields of health, recreation, dance, and physical education?

ans: Most of the people for whom they provide services

21-8 Why did AAHPER change from the American *Association* of HPER to the American *Alliance* of HPER?

ans: To represent the alliance of the various separate sub-groups and be an organization that was the "umbrella" that tied together the diverse fields that still maintain a common interest in sport

21-9 What has been one result of the rapid growth/development of recreation?

ans: It has moved from a base of primarily public services with many volunteer workers to a base of commercial/private services with paid workers.

21-10 What happens to professional preparation as a profession develops?

ans: The amount of professional preparation necessary to enter the profession increases.

21-11 What is the largest professional organization within the field of recreation?

ans: National Recreation and Park Association (NRPA)

21-12 What services are provided by the NRPA?

ans: a. Research
        b. Dissemination of program information
        c. Professional development
        d. Legislative policy information
        e. Field services to local groups
        f. Publications

21-13 What recreation association is affiliated with AAHPERD?

ans: American Association for Leisure and Recreation

21-14 How are licensing requirements typically set?

ans: State legislation establishes the work needed to earn certification.

21-15 Why do recreation programs offer accreditation in recreation?

ans: Accreditation ensures the public that personnel have competencies that cover safety and appropriate programming for recreational services.

21-16 What two fields could the area of stress management bring together?

ans: Recreation and health professions

21-17 If lifespan sport, fitness, and physical education are to become more of a reality for a larger percentage of the population, what must happen first?

ans: The interrelationships among the various fields will need to develop and strengthen.

21-18 On what does Johns (1985) feel that the future of people's health is dependent?

ans: What is done to promote, improve, and preserve the health of school- and college-age children and youth

21-19 To what approach have the health professions shifted, instead of the previous remedial approach?

ans: The preventative or "wellness" approach

21-20 What is the goal of the health enhancement industry?

ans: Improving the health of people

21-21 What has been the historical and present relationship of health to physical education?

ans: Health education used to be closely linked to the physical education curriculum and known as hygiene. It has, over the years, grown steadily more important and increasingly separate from physical education.

21-22 What is the most recent example of a social-medical problem that is being addressed by health educators?

ans: Acquired Immune Deficiency Syndrome (AIDS)

21-23 What are two examples of non-profit health organizations?

ans: a. The American Heart Association
        b. The Lung Association

21-24 What are the three main purposes of non-profit health associations?

ans: a. To generate financial support for research and program development in the
            particular area they serve
        b. To better educate the public about the central issues surrounding their focus
        c. To influence people to live better lifestyles

21-25 What sector in the health enhancement industry has experienced the strongest recent growth?

ans: Corporate and private sectors

21-26 According to Howe's (1983) estimation, what percentage of American corporations will provide employee recreation and fitness programs by 1990?

ans: 25%

21-27 What contributes to a certain amount of "quackery" in the private sector health enhancement industry?

ans: A combination of loosely regulated services and consumers who are anxious to improve but not always well informed about the services

21-28 What economic group of people have had little involvement in the wellness movement?

ans: Persons in lower income brackets with little discretionary income

21-29 What facts represent hope that Americans will decrease smoking habits?

ans: a. Fewer people smoke
        b. A smaller percentage start smoking

21-30 How widespread has dance been in the various cultures?

ans: Dance seems to be a significant human activity in virtually every culture known.

21-31 In what way was dance severely restricted in physical education programs?

ans: Whereas elementary physical educators might teach units in creative dance at the secondary level, folk dance was the only type of dance found with any frequency. Jazz or ballet were infrequent or impossible to find outside of private dance studios.

21-32 Why have physical educators been reluctant to teach dance?

ans: Few dance courses were required by their teacher preparation programs, so physical education majors frequently feel incapable of teaching dance.

21-33 What happened in the 1970s and 1980s to change the infrequency of dance programs?

ans: In the 1970s, dance began to be rediscovered as an important cultural form. In the educational reform climate of the 1980s, arts education has become a focus of school curriculum reform, and dance education has become part of an integrated arts approach in many elementary and middle schools.

21-34 Describe the movement known as "discipline-based arts education."

ans: The movement focuses on art as technique, but also has an equal emphasis on understanding the arts, becoming an educated, literate consumer of the arts, and being part of a knowledgeable arts audience.

21-35 What is involved in being a consumer of dance?

ans: Learning how to dance, how to create dances, how to make decisions about what they see in dance, and how to enjoy dance as a member of a dance audience

21-36 What two dance forms are the strongest at the university and college level?

ans: a. Ballet
        b. Modern

21-37 What has made dance more important in the elementary school curricula?

ans: a. Movement education
        b. The emerging integrated arts approach

21-38 Describe the current effects of the wellness revolution on children.

ans: Little effect—still low fitness levels, poor eating habits, and too much television.

Chapter 22

Sport, Fitness, and Physical Education in the Twenty-First Century: Themes Defining Our Future

True-False Questions

22-1 The Surgeon General's Report clearly established physical activity as a major public health issue.

22-2 Our professional capacity to meet the public-health challenge has been enhanced by our recent history of specialization.

22-3 Physical activity opportunities tend to be distributed equally across all socio-economic groups.

22-4 Research shows that computer technology has had an adverse affect on children's physical activity.

22-5 The primary benefit of the information technology age is better communication, storage, and reporting of data.

22-6 The age of hyperspecialization in both the academic disciplines of kinesiology and in professional physical education has outlived its usefulness.

22-7 Physical activity programs are part of a larger human-services profession.

22-8 Education and activity programs viewed as interventions to influence persons are studied by scholarly researchers rather than professionals.

22-9 In general, disciplinary research in physical education has informed the professional practice of physical education.

22-10 Disciplinarians have argued that a kinesiology curriculum provides the relevant foundation for professional study.

22-11 Activity and leisure services are being provided increasingly in the private sector.

22-12 Most leisure services involve user fees.

22-13 The activity and leisure industries have made a consistent effort to provide services for families in America that have marginal incomes.

22-14 Wellness has been accepted and encouraged by corporations because it increases the productivity of the workplace and reduces health costs.

22-15 At present, there is growing evidence that young persons across the income divisions of America are adopting a healthier lifestyle.

22-16 The sport culture of the United States tends to be exclusionary as children become youth and young adults.

22-17 Young adults typically do not engage in competitive sports.

22-18 Because of Title IX, women now have an equal share of facilities and budgets.

22-19 Many myths that serve to deter young girls from becoming involved in sport are social in origin but still lead to habits that reduce involvement.

22-20 The legal imperative of Title IX is more difficult to achieve than is the moral imperative that we eliminate gender prejudice from the culture.

22-21 Young children can be more easily educated and more easily directed in terms of lifestyle education than can adults, and at less cost.

22-22 We know more about the health and fitness status of children and youth than we do about young children or older adults.

22-23 A negative aspect to lifespan physical activity is that as people expend energy in physical activity they have less energy to do other things.

22-24 The focus of professional preparation programs will continue to need to be training people to work with school-age children.

True-False Answers

1. T	7. T	13. F	19. T
2. F	8. F	14. T	20. F
3. F	9. F	15. F	21. T
4. F	10. T	16. T	22. T
5 T	11. T	17. F	23. F
6. T	12. T	18. F	24. F

Short Answer Questions

22-1 In what ways does gender equity need to be promoted?

ans: Through legal means, through education

22-2 In what ways has information technology made a positive contribution to sport, fitness, and physical education?

ans: More information, information more accessible, storage and reporting of data, virtual exercise opportunities

22-3 Instead of physical education, what has the discipline movement tended to focus on?

ans: Sport and elite performers

22-4 Why has physical education tended to affiliate more and more with classroom research and practice rather than knowledge generated by the disciplines?

ans: The knowledge generated by the disciplines has tended to be theoretical with little practical application. Knowledge from classroom research is beneficial and applicable, so this has been the path taken.

22-5 What type of student will probably be attracted into the professional physical education program in the future?

ans: Those who want to teach and coach and those who want to work in the activity and leisure industry

22-6 What is the common characteristic of the activity and leisure services industry?

ans: Activity, both for health purposes and for leisure purposes

22-7 What is the status of regulation of the activity and service industry?

ans: It is largely unregulated, except as clients describe what programs they will support.

22-8 In the future, why can one expect more competition in the activity and leisure service industry?

ans: Because of the substantial amounts of money spent on the industry and the profits to be made

22-9 What has been the response of the sport, fitness, and physical education professions to the private sector industry?

ans: Except for programs in adult fitness, sport management, and recreation programs, they have not responded very quickly to the new industry. They still are preparing people primarily for employment in the public sector.

22-10 What is the professional obligation of those who are prepared with the knowledge and skill to provide appropriate activity programs for all ages?

ans: They should make this industry as good as it can be and inform citizens about the differences between good and bad programs instead of merely offering criticism.

22-11 What impact has the activity and leisure industry had on marginal income families in America?

ans: Very little

22-12 What has been the spending trend over the past quarter century for public expenditure on sport, fitness, and physical education?

ans: The trend has been to reduce public spending, making access to opportunity in sport, fitness, and physical education increasingly tied to wealth.

22-13 What components are included in the wellness component?

ans: a. Nutrition
         b. Body image
         c. Emotional well-being
         d. Stress management
         e. Spiritual wellness

22-14 What benefits would there be with the adoption of a wellness lifestyle by the larger population?

ans: a. Increase the productivity of work places
         b. Reduce the staggering costs of health and medical care

22-15 What is an important component of the wellness philosophy?

ans: That individuals should take responsibility for their own health and lifestyle

22-16 What is the net result of the socially invented myths surrounding females in sport and fitness?

ans: They have tended to exclude girls and women from the opportunity to participate. These habits may persist to adulthood.

22-17 What is consumer education and why is it important to the wellness movement?

ans: Consumer education teaches the public to choose products and services because of their benefits, rather than based on fads or false information. Currently, profit is dictating practice. The public needs to be educated about products and services and their contribution to healthy living.

22-18 Where does lifestyle education need to begin? Why?

ans: It needs to begin with the very young children and is most important in elementary and middle school, when habits form and children adopt activity patterns that often last a lifetime.

22-19 What are two ways in which the problem of sport, fitness, and physical education only for those people with discretionary income can be addressed?

ans: a. Redistribute the income more equitably across the economic classes
        b. Distribute programs more through the public sector

22-20 Why is the varsity model not as receptive to lifespan sport as the European club model?

ans: The varsity model tends to be exclusionary and only the best participate as children get older. In the European club model, athletes can join clubs as youngsters and compete in organized competition at their own level of development for as long as they want.

22-21 Why is acquisition of strong "people" skills going to be important for young fitness and sport professionals?

ans: People attend fitness spas for social reasons as well as fitness ones. Teaching in physical education and fitness programs will require a high personal touch or a high degree of interpersonal attention, and new trainees must learn how to provide this need as well as being proficient in their areas.

22-22 What is even more important than legislation such as Title IX?

ans: There is a moral imperative to rid our culture of prejudices against girls and women. Sport, fitness, and physical education professionals need to be advocates for girls and women.

22-23 What three changes in school physical education are necessary to reverse the current trends and prevent its demise?

ans: a. Students must get and stay fit.
       b. Students need to learn the skills and strategies of sports and enjoy playing them.
       c. Students should develop strong and independent leisure skills.

22-24 To which age groups does the focus of our profession need to expand?

ans: a. To those younger than kindergarten
       b. To the post-college adult, all the way to programs for senior citizens

22-25 What knowledge and skills different from those typically included in a professional preparation program will be necessary for an expanded physical education/fitness/sport program?

ans: a. How to work with the new age groups
       b. How to service the private vs. public sector

Essay Questions, Class Activities, and Student Projects

Suggestions for essay questions, class activities, and student projects are listed below by chapter. Most of the suggestions, however, could easily be used in alternative ways; that is, a suggested class activity in the form of a debate could easily be made into an essay question or into class discussion activity. Suggestions described as projects could easily become essay questions or class activities.

For example, one of the suggested debate topics focuses on coaching requirements.

Debate: Resolved, adults who coach children's sport teams should be required to complete a minimum certification similar to the ASEP Volunteer level. Choose three-person student teams to argue the affirmative and negative.

This debate could easily be made into an essay question.

Essay: State and defend a position which either supports or rejects the following proposition: Adults who coach children's sport teams should be required to complete a minimum certification similar to the ASEP Volunteer level.

The issue could also be organized as a class project.

Project: Make contact with a children's sport program. Find out how coaches are recruited and what training, if any, they are required to complete before they are approved to coach. Observe coaches during a practice session. Assess the degree to which they interact with children in ways that are consistent with what is suggested in the ASEP Volunteer level coaching guide. Write a 2–3 page report describing what you found.

Chapter 1.   Lifespan, Sport, Fitness, and Physical Education

Project or class activity: Have students reflect on the physical activity interests and habits of their parents and grandparents. Were there gender differences? Was age stereotyping evident?

Project: Have students visit local agencies, clubs, and organizations that sponsor physical activity programs. Students can report on who participates, what programs are available, and what the costs are.

Chapter 2.   The Emergence of a Profession: 1885–1930

Essay: Describe how physical education and sport emerged from different forces in the latter half of the 19th century.

Debate: Resolved, the stereotyping of gender roles in current sport and physical activity participation is merely a modified version of the masculinity/femininity expectations of the 19th century.

Chapter 3.   Consolidation and Specialization: 1930–Present

Project or class activity: Have students examine and discuss the various degree programs in the department for the influence of the discipline movement.

Project: Have students gather information to report on the structure, membership, and purposes of important professional organizations such as ACSM, AAHPERD, NASPE, NAPEHE, and NRPA.

Chapter 4.   Changing Philosophies for Sport, Fitness, and Physical Education

Discussion, essay, or class activity: Have students examine various sports and compare the ideal of fair play as it is or is not practiced in the sport. Suggested sports are golf, tennis, ice hockey, American football, track and field, and field hockey.

Debate: Resolved, sport participation does contribute to the positive development of character.

Essay: Take a position for or against the following assertion and defend the position: There are no women's sports in America, only men's sports in which women participate.

Chapter 5.   Basic Concepts of Sport

Essay: Define the concepts of leisure, play, and games, and explain how each relates to sport.

Discussion/essay: Explain and provide examples of the three meanings of competition.

Debate: Resolved, ultimate Frisbee is not a sport.

Class activity: Divide the class into four groups. Assign each group a game classification. Each member of the group chooses one game in that classification and identifies and explains the primary and secondary rules for that game.

Chapter 6. Sport Programs and Professions

Class activity: Divide the class into three groups. Assign groups to children's, interscholastic, or intercollegiate sport. Groups discuss important issues for that level of sport and present a list of the five most important issues to the remainder of the class.

Debate or essay: Resolved, the varsity model of interscholastic sport in the USA is superior to the club model in Europe.

Project: Have each student choose a nonparticipant sport vocation. They must investigate the requirements for that vocation, likely entry pay, and career possibilities. Present to class or write a short paper.

Chapter 7. Problems and Issues in Sport

Essay: Take and defend a position on the question of how early young athletes should be allowed to specialize in year-round training.

Essay or class activity: Identify a specific equity issue in youth or school sport from the students' experiences. Suggest possible solutions and decide on the best suggestion.

Debate: Resolved, eligibility rules for sport participation discriminate against less academically talented students and should be abolished so that any student in good standing in the school could participate.

Chapter 8. Basic Concepts of Fitness

Debate: Resolved, physical fitness testing in school PE should be eliminated.

Essay: Take and defend a point of view on which approach to the dose-response debate is most appropriate for school PE.

Project: Have each student attend and observe a fitness session of some kind (strength room in school, aerobics session, fitness club, etc.). Have them report on who is participating and what kind of fitness the activity promotes.

Chapter 9. Fitness Programs and Professions

Project: Have students prepare a memoir of their fitness experiences in school PE and evaluate those experiences in terms of the quality programs described in this chapter.

Essay: Describe the various opportunities for a career in the fitness professions.

Debate: Resolved, school PE should focus solely on health-related PE.

Chapter 10. Problems and Issues in Fitness

Essay: Describe and provide examples of what is meant by an infrastructure to support lifetime physical activity.

Project: Have students prepare a description of a model fitness-oriented school PE program that does not require more resources than most schools can afford.

Class activity: Divide the class into four teams. Give the same four "fitness problems" to each team and have them arrive at a preferred solution. Then, have the teams compare and discuss their solutions.

Chapter 11. Basic Concepts of Physical Education

Essay: Discuss how concerns over liability have had a positive and negative influence on physical education.

Debate: Resolved, all students with disabilities should be included in regular physical education classes.

Project or essay: Develop a set of objectives that you believe best define a quality physical education and describe the kind of program you might develop to achieve those objectives.

Chapter 12. Physical Education Programs and Professions

Essay or project: Describe the common characteristics of physical education programs that work and compare them to the high school physical education program you experienced.

Class activity: Divide the class into four teams. Assign each of them a program model and have the team describe how they would implement the model in a local elementary or high school.

Debate: Resolved, there should be a national physical education program that defines what is done at each grade level in physical education.

Chapter 13. Problems and Issues in Physical Education

Debate: Competition should be eliminated from elementary physical education programs.

Class activity: Divide the class into working groups. Assign each the same task: How would you build the credibility of a high school PE program and communicate the benefits of the program to the local community?

Essay or project: Describe how you would develop a school PE program that allowed students of differing skill levels to learn and perform together.

Chapter 14. Exercise Physiology

Essay: Describe the field of exercise physiology and why it is important to the fitness professions.

Chapter 15. Kinesiology and Biomechanics

Essay: Describe how kinesiology and biomechanics have made positive contributions to both daily living and elite sport performance.

Chapter 16. Motor Learning, Control, and Development

Project: Have students visit a local physical activity program for young children (Gymboree, etc.) and report their observations of what goes on in the program.

Chapter 17. Sport Sociology

Essay or project: Have students examine the social class structure of sport spectating. Which sport contests appeal to various classes? What are the characteristics of those sports?

Chapter 18.   Sport Psychology

Project: Have each student examine their own sport experience and describe the aspects of their experience where psychological problems were possible or psychological interventions might have been helpful.

Chapter 19.   Sport Pedagogy

Class activity: Divide the class into four teams. Assign two teams the topic of pedagogy for coaching preparation and two teams the topic of pedagogy for teacher preparation. Have each team define what they see as the most important content and experiences that should be included in the preparation program.

Chapter 20.   The Sport Humanities

Class activity or project: Show a sport film in class or assign students to watch it on a video rental. Have them discuss or write a paper analyzing what the film says about the meaning and influence of sport. Suggested films would be Chariots of Fire, The Bad News Bears, or Field of Dreams.

Chapter 21.   Relationships to Allied Fields

Essay: Describe the differences between a medical-remedial approach to health and a wellness or lifestyle approach.

Project: Have students investigate all the physical activity program opportunities for children and youth in their local area with a focus on what agencies provide the opportunities. Have them comment on the degree to which the separation of health, dance, recreation, and physical education hinders or helps to contribute to a coherent set of program opportunities.

Debate: Resolved, the fields of health, recreation, dance, and physical education should remain separate and distinct to allow for their further development and professional identity.

Chapter 22.   Sport, Fitness, and Physical Education in the Twenty-First Century: Themes Defining Our Future

Project: Have each student choose a theme and write an editorial stating and defending a position related to the theme.

Debate: Resolved, the social gradient in health and leisure demands that the federal government institute programs that serve the poor and working classes.

Class activity: Put each theme on a slip of paper. Have students come forward and choose a slip of paper from a container. They then have to speak directly to a preferred outcome for the theme; that is, what should happen and what needs to be done to make it happen. Give students a few moments to compose their responses.